Eat Right 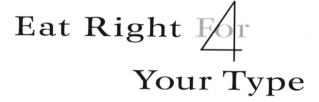 For 4
Your Type

DR. PETER J. D'ADAMO

WITH CATHERINE WHITNEY

G. P. PUTNAM'S SONS
NEW YORK

4 BLOOD TYPES,
4 DIETS

Eat Right For *Your* Type

The Individualized
Diet Solution
to Staying Healthy,
Living Longer &
Achieving Your Ideal Weight

G. P. Putnam's Sons
Publishers Since 1838
a member of
Penguin Putnam Inc.
375 Hudson Street
New York, NY 10014

Library of Congress Cataloging-in-Publication Data

D'Adamo, Peter. Eat right 4 your type: the individualized diet
solution to staying healthy, living longer and achieving your
ideal weight / Peter D'Adamo, with Catherine Whitney.
p. cm.
Includes index.
ISBN 0-399-14255-X
1. Blood groups. 2. Nutrition. 3. Health. 4. Weight loss.
5. Human evolution. I. Whitney, Catherine (Catherine A.)
II. Title.
QP98.D33   1996   96-35510 CIP
613—dc20

Printed in the United States of America
100

This book is printed on acid-free paper. ∞

BOOK DESIGN BY DEBORAH KERNER

To the memory of my good friend,
JOHN J. MOSKO (1919–1992)

"This day is called the feast of Crispian:
He that outlives this day, and comes home safe,
Will stand a tip-toe when this day is named,
And rouse him at the name of Crispian."

Acknowledgments

THERE ARE MANY PEOPLE TO THANK, AS NO SCIENTIFIC pursuit is solitary. Along the way, I have been driven, inspired, and supported by all of the people who placed their confidence in me. In particular, I give deep thanks to my wife, Martha Mosko D'Adamo, for her love and friendship; my parents, James D'Adamo Sr., N.D., and Christiana, for teaching me to trust in my intuition; and my brother, James D'Adamo Jr., for believing in me.

I am also more grateful than I can express to:

Joseph Pizzorno, N.D., for inspiring me to trust in the science of natural medicine;

Catherine Whitney, my writer, who imparted a style and organization to the raw material characteristic of a true wordsmith;

Gail Winston, the editor who long ago, out of the clear blue sky, rang me up and asked me if I wanted to write a book about natural medicine;

My literary agent, Janis Vallely, who saw the promise of my work and didn't allow it to languish somewhere in a dusty file cabinet;

Amy Hertz, my editor at Riverhead/Putnam, whose vision turned the manuscript into the rich and important document I believe it has now become.

I am also thankful to:

Dorothy Mosko, for her invaluable assistance in the preparation of the early manuscript;

Scott Carlson, my erstwhile assistant, who never missed a UPS pickup;

Carolyn Knight, R.N., my right-hand nurse and expert phlebotomist;

Jane Dystel, Catherine's literary agent, whose advice was always on target;

Paul Krafin, who lent his sharp writing and editing skills to the revision process;

Dina Khader, R.D., who helped with the recipes and meal planning;

Michael Schachter, M.D., Jonathan Wright, M.D., and Alan Datner, M.D., for their valuable suggestions and guidance.

John Schuler, who designed the illustrations.

I also wish to thank the research interns at Bastyr University, who expertly sifted through the extensive medical literature pertaining to blood type, helping to make this book as complete an account of the subject as possible.

Lastly, I thank all the wonderful patients, who in their quest for health and happiness chose to honor me with their trust.

Contents

The Work
of Two Lives

I believed that no two people on the face of the earth were alike; no two people have the same fingerprints, lip prints, or voice prints. No two blades of grass or snowflakes are alike. Because I felt that all people were different from one another, I did not think it was logical that they should eat the same foods. It became clear to me that since each person was housed in a special body with different strengths, weaknesses, and nutritional requirements, the only way to maintain health or cure illness was to accommodate to that particular patient's specific needs.

James D'Adamo,
my father

YOUR BLOOD TYPE IS THE KEY THAT UNLOCKS THE DOOR to the mysteries of health, disease, longevity, physical vitality, and emotional strength. Your blood type determines your susceptibility to illness, which foods you should eat, and how you should exercise. It is a factor in your energy levels, in the efficiency with which you "burn" calories, in your emotional response to stress, and perhaps even in your personality.

The connection between blood type and diet may sound radical, but it is not. We have long known that there was a missing link in our comprehension of the process that leads either to the path of wellness or to the dismal trail of disease. There had to be a reason why there were so many paradoxes in dietary studies and disease survival. There also had to be an explanation for why some people were able to lose weight on particular diets, while others were not; why some people retained vitality late in life, while others deteriorated mentally and physically. Blood type analysis has given us a way to explain these paradoxes. And the more we explore the connection, the more valid it becomes.

Blood types are as fundamental as creation itself. In the masterly logic of nature, blood types follow an unbroken trail from the earliest moment of human creation to the present day. They are the signature of our ancient ancestors on the indestructible parchment of history.

Now we have begun to discover how to use the blood type as a cellular fingerprint that unravels many of the major mysteries surrounding our quest for good health. This work is an extension of the recent groundbreaking findings concerning human DNA. Our understanding of blood type takes the science of genetics one step further by stating unequivocally that every human being is utterly unique. There is no right or wrong lifestyle or diet; there are only right or wrong choices to be made based on our individual genetic codes.

How I Found the Missing Blood Type Link

MY WORK in the field of blood type analysis is the fulfillment of a lifetime pursuit—not only my own but also my father's. I am a second-generation naturopathic physician. Dr. James D'Adamo, my father, graduated from naturopathic college (a four-year postgraduate program) in 1957 and later studied in Europe at several of the great spas. He noticed that although many patients did well on strict vegetarian and low-fat diets, which are the hallmarks of "spa cuisine," a certain number of patients did not appear to improve, and some did poorly or even worsened. A sensitive man with keen powers of deduction and insight, my father reasoned that there should be some sort of blueprint that he could use to determine differences in the dietary needs of his patients. He rationalized that since blood was the fundamental source of nourishment to the body, perhaps some aspect of the blood could help identify these differences. My father set about testing this theory by blood-typing his patients and observing individualized reactions when they were prescribed different diets.

Through the years and with countless patients, a pattern began to emerge. He noticed that patients who were Type A seemed to do poorly on high-protein diets that included generous portions of meat, but did very well on vegetable proteins such as soy and tofu. Dairy products tended to produce copious amounts of mucous discharge in the sinuses and respiratory passages of Type As. When told to increase their levels of physical activity and exercise, Type As usually felt fatigued and unwell; when they performed lighter forms of exercise, such as yoga, they felt alert and energized.

On the other hand, Type O patients thrived on high-protein diets, and they felt invigorated by intense physical activities, such as jogging and aerobics. The more my father tested the different blood types, the greater his conviction became that each of them followed a distinct path to wellness.

Inspired by the saying "One man's food is another man's poison," my father condensed his observations and dietary recommendations into a book he titled *One Man's Food*. When the book was published in 1980, I was in my third year of naturopathic studies at Seattle's John Bastyr College. During this time revolutionary gains were being achieved in naturopathic education. The goal of Bastyr College was nothing less than to produce the complete alternative physician, the intellectual and scientific equal of a medical internist, but with specialized naturopathic training. For the first time naturopathic techniques, procedures, and substances could be scientifically evaluated with the benefits of modern technology. I waited for an opportunity to research my father's blood type theory. I wanted to assure myself that it carried valid scientific weight. My chance came in 1982, my senior year, when, for a clinical rounds requirement, I began scanning the medical literature to see if I could find any correlation between the ABO blood types and a predilection for certain diseases, and whether any of this supported my father's diet theory. Since my father's book was based on his subjective impressions of the blood types rather than on an objective method of evaluation, I wasn't certain that I would be able to find any scientific basis for his theories. But I was amazed at what I learned.

My first breakthrough came with the discovery that two major diseases of the stomach were associated with blood type. The first was the peptic ulcer, a condition often related to higher-than-average stomach-acid levels. This condition was reported to be more common in people with Type O blood than in people with other blood types. I was immediately intrigued, since my father had observed that Type O patients did well on animal products and protein diets—foods that require more stomach acid for proper digestion.

The second correlation was an association between Type A and stomach cancer. Stomach cancer was often linked to low levels of stomach-acid production, as was pernicious anemia, another disorder found more often in Type A individuals. Pernicious anemia is related to a lack of vitamin B-12, which requires sufficient stomach acid for its absorption.

As I studied these facts I realized that on the one hand, Type O blood predisposed people to an illness associated with too much stomach acid, while on the other hand, Type A blood predisposed people to two illnesses associated with too little stomach acid.

That was the link I'd been looking for. There absolutely was a scientific basis for my father's observations. And so began my ongoing love affair with the science and anthropology of the blood types. In time, I found that my father's initial work on the correlation between blood type, diet and health was far more significant than even he had imagined.

Four Simple Keys to Unlock Life's Mysteries

I GREW UP in a family that was mostly Blood Type A, and because of my father's work we ate a basically vegetarian diet consisting of foods such as tofu, steamed vegetables, and salads. As a child I was often embarrassed and felt somewhat deprived, because none of my friends ate weird foods like tofu. To the contrary, they were happily engaged in another kind of "diet revolution" sweeping the 1950s; their diets consisted of hamburgers, hot dogs, greasy french fries, candy bars, ice cream, and lots of soda pop.

Today, I still eat the way I did as a child, and I love it. Every day I eat the foods that my Type A body craves, and it's immensely satisfying.

In *Eat Right 4 Your Type* I will teach you about the fundamental relationship between your blood type and the dietary and lifestyle choices that will help you live at your very best. The essence of the blood type connection rests in these facts:

- Your blood type—O, A, B, or AB—is a powerful genetic fingerprint that identifies you as surely as your DNA.
- When you use the individualized characteristics of your blood type as a guidepost for eating and living, you will be healthier, you will naturally reach your ideal weight, and you will slow the process of aging.
- Your blood type is a more reliable measure of your identity than race, culture, or geography. It is a genetic blueprint for who you are, a guide to how you can live most healthfully.
- The key to the significance of blood type can be found in the story of human evolution: Type O is the oldest; Type A evolved with agrarian society; Type B emerged as humans migrated north into colder, harsher territories; and Type AB was a thoroughly modern adaptation, a result of the intermingling of disparate groups. This evolutionary story relates directly to the dietary needs of each blood type today.

What is this remarkable factor, the blood type?

Blood type is one of several medically recognized variations, much like hair and eye color. Many of these variations, such as fingerprint patterns and the more recent DNA analysis, are used extensively by forensic scientists and criminalists, as well as those who research the causes and cures of disease. Blood type is every bit as significant as other variations; in many ways, it's a more useful measure. Blood type analysis is a logical system. The information is simple to learn and easy to follow. I've taught the system to numerous doctors, who tell me they are getting good results with patients who follow its guidelines. Now I will teach it to you. By learning the principles of blood type analysis, you can tailor the optimal diet for yourself and your family members. You can pinpoint the foods that make you sick, contribute to weight gain, and lead to chronic disease.

Early on, I realized that blood type analysis offered a powerful means of interpreting individual variations in health and disease. Given the amount of available research data, it is surprising that the effects of blood type on our health have not received the measure of attention that they deserve. But now I am prepared to make that information available—not just to my fellow scientists and colleagues in the medical community, but to you.

At first glance, the science of blood type may seem daunting, but I assure you it is as simple and basic as life itself. I will tell you about the ancient trail of the evolution of blood types (as riveting as the story of human history), and demystify the science of blood types to provide a clear and simple plan that you will be able to follow.

I realize that this is probably a completely new idea for you. Few people ever even think about the implications of their blood type, even though it is a powerful genetic force. You may be reluctant to wade into such unfamiliar territory, even if the scientific arguments seem convincing. I ask you to do only three things: Talk to your physician before you begin, find out your blood type if you don't already know it, and try your Blood Type Diet for at least two weeks. Most of my patients experience some results within that time period—increased energy, weight loss, a lessening of digestive complaints, and improvement of chronic problems such as asthma, headaches, and heartburn. Give your

Blood Type Diet a chance to bring you the benefits I've seen it bring to the more than four thousand people I've put on the diet. See for yourself that blood not only provides your body's most vital nourishment, but now proves itself a vehicle for your future well-being.

Your Blood Type Identity

Blood Type:

The Real
Evolution Revolution

LOOD IS LIFE ITSELF. IT IS THE PRIMAL FORCE that fuels the power and mystery of birth, the horrors of disease, war, and violent death. Entire civilizations have been built on blood ties. Tribes, clans, and monarchies depend on them. We cannot exist without blood—literally or figuratively.

Blood is magical. Blood is mystical. Blood is alchemical. It appears throughout human history as a profound religious and cultural symbol. Ancient peoples mixed it together and drank it to denote unity and fealty. From the earliest times, hunters performed rituals to appease the spirits of the animals they killed by offering up the animal blood and smearing it on their faces and bodies. The blood of the lamb was placed as a mark on the hovels of the enslaved Jews of Egypt so that the Angel of Death would pass over them. Moses is said to have turned the waters of Egypt to blood in his quest to free his people. The symbolic blood of Jesus Christ has been, for nearly two thousand years, central to the most sacred rite of Christianity.

Blood evokes such rich and sacred imagery because it is in reality so extraordinary. Not only does it supply the complex delivery and defense systems that are necessary for our very existence, it provides a keystone for humanity—a looking glass through which we can trace the faint tracks of our journey.

In the last forty years we have been able to use biological markers such as blood type to map the movements and groupings of our ancestors. By learning how these early people adapted to the challenges posed by constantly changing climates, germs, and diets, we are learning about ourselves. Change in climate and available food produced new blood types. Blood type is the unbroken cord that binds us to one another.

Ultimately, the differences in blood types reflect upon the human ability to acclimate to different environmental challenges. For the most part, these challenges impacted the digestive and immune systems: a piece of bad meat could kill you; a cut or scrape could evolve into a deadly infection. Yet the human race survived. And the story of that survival is inextricably tied to our digestive and immune systems. It is in these two areas that most of the distinctions between blood types are found.

The Human Story

THE STORY OF humankind is the story of survival. More specifically, it is the story of where humans lived and what they could eat there. It is about food—about finding food and moving to find food. We don't know for certain when the human evolution began. Neanderthals, the first humanoids we can recognize, may have developed 500,000 years ago. Maybe more.

We do know that human prehistory began in Africa, where we evolved from humanlike creatures. Early life was short, nasty, and brutish. People died a thousand different ways—opportunistic infections, parasites, animal attacks, broken bones, childbirth—and they died young.

Early humans must have had a harrowing time providing for themselves in this savage environment. Their teeth were short and blunt—ill suited for attack. Unlike most of their competitors on the food chain, they had no special abilities with regard to speed, strength, or agility. Initially, the chief quality humans possessed was an innate cunning, which later grew to reasoned thought.

Neanderthals probably ate a rather crude diet of wild plants, grubs, and the scavenged leftovers from the kills of predatory animals. They were more prey than predator, especially when it came to infections and parasitic afflictions. (Many of the parasites, worms, flukes, and infectious microorganisms found in Africa do not stimulate the immune system to produce a specific antibody to them, probably because the early Type O people already had protection in the form of the antibodies they carried from birth.)

As the human race moved around and was forced to adapt its diet to changing conditions, the new diet provoked adaptations in the digestive tract and immune system necessary for it to first survive and later thrive in each new habitat. These changes are reflected in the development of the blood types, which appear to have arrived at critical junctures of human development:

1. The ascent of humans to the top of the food chain (evolution of Type O to its fullest expression).
2. The change from hunter-gatherer to a more domesticated agrarian lifestyle (appearance of Type A).
3. The merging and migration of the races from the African homeland to Europe, Asia, and the Americas (development of Type B).
4. The modern intermingling of disparate groups (the arrival of Type AB).

Each blood type contains the genetic message of our ancestors' diets and behaviors, and though we're a long way away from early history, many of their traits still affect us. Knowing these predispositions helps us to understand the logic of the blood type diets.

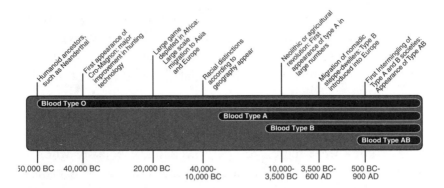

The blood type–anthropology timeline. Starting from earliest times, the diagram highlights various human developments in relation to the introduction of the blood types. Interestingly, the evolutionary changes in blood type have almost a biblical time frame. When everyone was Type O (the longest period of time), and they occupied a contracted living space, ate the same diet, and breathed in the same organisms, any further change was unnecessary. However, with the increase in population and subsequent migrations, variation accelerated. The subsequent Blood Types A and B are no more than 15,000 to 25,000 years old, and Type AB is far more recent.

O Is for Old

THE APPEARANCE of our Cro-Magnon ancestors in around 40,000
B.C. propelled the human species to the top of the food chain,
making them the most dangerous predators on earth. They began to hunt in organized packs; in a short time, they were able
to make weapons and use tools. These major advances gave
them strength and superiority beyond their natural physical
abilities.

Skillful and formidable hunters, the Cro-Magnons soon had
little to fear from any of their animal rivals. With no natural predators other than themselves, the population exploded. Protein—
meat—was their fuel, and it was at this point that the digestive
attributes of Blood Type O reached their fullest expression.

Humans thrived on meat, and it took a remarkably short time
for them to kill off the big game within their hunting range.
There were more and more people to feed, so competition for

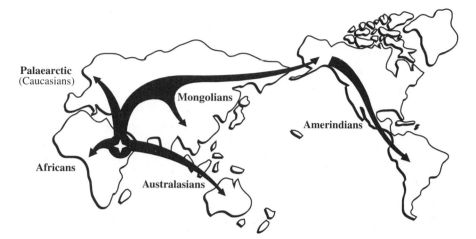

From their base in the ancestral homeland of Africa, early Blood Type O hunter-gatherers wandered throughout Africa and into Europe and Asia in search of new supplies of large game. As they encountered changing environmental conditions, they began to develop modern racial characteristics.

meat became intense. Hunters began fighting and killing others who were impinging on what they claimed were their exclusive hunting grounds. As always, human beings found their greatest enemy to be themselves. Good hunting areas became scarce. The migration of the human race began.

By 30,000 B.C., bands of hunters were traveling farther and farther in search of meat. When a shift in the trade winds desiccated what had been fertile hunting land in the African Sahara, and when previously frozen northern areas grew warmer, they began to move out of Africa into Europe and Asia.

This movement seeded the planet with its base population, which was Blood Type O, the predominant blood type even today.

By 20,000 B.C. Cro-Magnons had moved fully into Europe and Asia, decimating the vast herds of large game to such an extent that other foods had to be found. Searching each new area for anything edible, it is likely that the carnivorous humans quickly became omnivorous, with a mixed diet of berries, grubs, nuts, roots, and small animals. Populations also thrived along the coastlines and the teeming lakes and rivers of the earth where fish and other food were abundant. By 10,000 B.C., humans occupied every main landmass on the planet, except for Antarctica.

The movement of the early humans to less temperate climates created lighter skins, less massive bone structures, and straighter hair. Nature, over time, reacclimated them to the regions of the earth they inhabited. People moved northward, so light skin developed, which was better protected against frostbite than dark skin. Lighter skin was also better able to metabolize vitamin D in a land of shorter days and longer nights.

The Cro-Magnons eventually burned themselves out; their success was anathema. Overpopulation soon exhausted the available hunting grounds. What had once seemed like an unending supply of large game animals diminished sharply. This led to increased competition for the remaining meat. Competition led to war, and war to further migration.

A Is for Agrarian

T YPE A BLOOD initially appeared somewhere in Asia or the Middle East between 25,000 and 15,000 B.C. in response to new environmental conditions. It emerged at the peak of the Neolithic period, or New Stone Age, which followed the Old Stone Age, or Paleolithic period, of the Cro-Magnon hunters. Agriculture and animal domestication were the hallmarks of its culture.

The cultivation of grains and livestock changed everything. Able to forgo their hand-to-mouth existence and sustain themselves for the first time, people established stable communities and permanent living structures. This radically different lifestyle, a major change in diet and environment, resulted in an entirely new mutation in the digestive tracts and the immune systems of the Neolithic peoples—a mutation that allowed them to better tolerate and absorb cultivated grains and other agricultural products. Type A was born.

Settling into permanent farming communities presented new developmental challenges. The skills necessary for hunting together now gave way to a different kind of cooperative society. For the first time, a specific skill at doing one thing depended on the skills of others doing something else. For example, the miller depended on the farmer to bring in his crops; the farmer depended on the miller to grind his grain. One no longer thought of food as only an immediate source of nourishment or as a sometime thing. Fields needed to be sown and cultivated in anticipation of future reward. Planning and networking with others became the order of the day. Psychologically, these are traits at which Type As excel—perhaps another environmental adaptation.

The gene for Type A began to thrive in the early agrarian societies. The genetic mutation that produced Type A from Type O occurred rapidly—so rapidly that the rate of mutation was comparable to four times that of *Drosophila*, the common fruit fly and current record holder!

What could have been the reason for this extraordinary rate of human mutation from Type O to Type A? It was survival. Survival of the fittest in a crowded society. Because Type A emerged as more resistant to infections common to densely populated areas, urban, industrialized societies quickly became Type A. Even today, survivors of plague, cholera, and smallpox show a predominance of Type A over Type O.

Eventually, the gene for Type A blood spread beyond Asia and the Middle East into western Europe, carried by the Indo-Europeans, who penetrated deeply into the pre-Neolithic populations. The Indo-European hordes originally appeared in south-central Russia, and between 3,500 and 2,000 B.C. pushed southward into the top of southwestern Asia, creating the populations and peoples of Iran and Afghanistan. Ever burgeoning, they moved further westward into Europe. The Indo-European invasion was really the original Diet Revolution. It introduced new foods and lifestyle habits into the simpler immune systems and digestive tracts of the early hunter-gatherers, and those changes were so profound that they produced the environmental stress necessary to spread the Type A gene. In time, the digestive system of the hunter-gatherers lost its ability to digest its carnivorous pre-agricultural diet.

Today, Type A blood is still found in its highest concentration among western Europeans. The frequency of Type A diminishes as we head eastward from western Europe, following the receding trails of the ancient migratory patterns. Type A peoples are highly concentrated across the Mediterranean, Adriatic, and Aegean seas, particularly in Corsica, Sardinia, Spain, Turkey, and the Balkans. The Japanese also have some of the highest concentrations of Type As in eastern Asia, along with a moderately high number of blood Type Bs.

Blood Type A had mutated from Type O in response to the myriad infections provoked by an increased populace and major dietary changes. But Blood Type B was different.

B Is for Balance

BLOOD TYPE B developed sometime between 10,000 and 15,000 B.C., in the area of the Himalayan highlands—now part of present-day Pakistan and India.

Pushed from the hot, lush savannahs of eastern Africa to the cold, unyielding highlands of the Himalayas, Blood Type B may have initially mutated in response to climactic changes. It first appeared in India or the Ural region of Asia among a mix of Caucasian and Mongolian tribes. This new blood type was soon characteristic of the great tribes of steppe dwellers, who by this time dominated the Eurasian plains.

As the Mongolians swept through Asia, the gene for Type B blood was firmly entrenched. The Mongolians spread northward, pursuing a culture dependent upon herding and domesticating animals—as their diet of meat and cultured dairy products reflected.

Two distinct Type Bs sprang up as the pastoral nomads pushed into Asia: an agrarian, comparatively sedentary group in the south and the east; and a nomadic, warlike society conquering the north and the west. The nomads were expert horsemen who penetrated far into eastern Europe, and the gene for Type B blood is

Origins and movements of Type A and Type B. From its beginnings in Asia and the Middle East, the gene for Type A was carried by Indo-European peoples into western and northern Europe. Other migrations carried Type A into northern Africa, where it spread into the Saharan Africans. From its origins in the western Himalayan mountains, Type B was carried by Mongolian peoples into southeast Asia and into the Asian flatlands or steppes. A separate migration of Type B peoples entered eastern Europe. By this time the sea levels of the earth had risen, removing the land bridge between North America and Asia. This prevented any movement of Type B into North America, where the earlier populations continued on as exclusively Type O.

---

still in strong evidence in many of the eastern European populations. In the meantime, an entire agriculturally based culture had spread throughout China and southeast Asia. Because of the nature of the land they chose to till, and climates unique to their areas, these peoples created and employed sophisticated irrigation and cultivation techniques that displayed an awesome blend of creativity, intelligence, and engineering.

The schism between the warlike tribes to the north and the peaceful farmers to the south was deep, and its remnants exist to this day in southern Asian cuisine, which uses little if any dairy foods. To the Asian mind, dairy products are the food of the barbarian, which is unfortunate because the diet they have adopted does not suit Type Bs as well.

Of all the ABO types, Type B shows the most clearly defined geographic distribution. Stretching as a great belt across the Eurasian plains and down to the Indian subcontinent, Type B is found in increased numbers from Japan, Mongolia, China, and India up to the Ural Mountains. From there westward, the percentages fall until a low is reached at the western tip of Europe.

The small numbers of Type B in Old and Western Europeans represents western migration by Asian nomadic peoples. This is best seen in the easternmost western Europeans, the Germans and Austrians, who have an unexpectedly high incidence of Type B blood compared to their western neighbors. The highest occurrence of Type B in Germans occurs in the area around the upper and middle Elbe River, which had been nominally held as the dividing line between civilization and barbarism in ancient times.

Modern subcontinental Indians, a Caucasian people, have some of the highest frequencies of Type B blood in the world. The northern Chinese and Koreans have very high rates of Type B blood and very low rates of Type A.

The blood type characteristics of the various Jewish populations have long been of interest to anthropologists. As a general rule, regardless of their nationality or race, there is a trend toward higher-than-average rates of Type B blood. The Ashkenazim and the Sephardim, the two major Jewish sects, share strong levels of Type B blood, and appear to have very few differences. The pre-Diaspora Babylonian Jews differ considerably from the primarily Type O Arabic population of Iraq (the location of the biblical Babylon) in that they are primarily Type B, with some frequency of Type A.

AB Is for Modern

TYPE AB BLOOD is rare. Emerging from the intermingling of Type A Caucasians with Type B Mongolians, it is found in less than 5 percent of the population, and it is the newest of the blood types.

Until ten or twelve centuries ago, there was no Type AB blood. Then barbarian hordes sliced through the soft underbelly of many collapsing civilizations, overrunning the length and breadth of the Roman Empire. As a result of the intermingling of these Eastern invaders with the last trembling vestiges of European civilization, Type AB blood came to be. No evidence for the occurrence of this blood type extends beyond nine hundred to a thousand years ago, when a large western migration of eastern peoples took place. Blood Type AB is rarely found in European graves prior to A.D. 900. Studies on exhumations of prehistoric graves in Hungary show a distinct lack of this blood group into the Longobard age (fourth to seventh century A.D.). This would seem to indicate that up until that point in time, European populations of Type A and Type B did not come into common contact, or if so, did not mingle or intermarry.

Because Type ABs inherit the tolerance of both Type A and Type B, their immune systems have an enhanced ability to manufacture more specific antibodies to microbial infections. This unique quality of possessing neither anti-A nor anti-B antibodies minimizes their chances of being prone to allergies and other autoimmune diseases such as arthritis, inflammation, and lupus. There is, however, a greater predisposition to certain cancers because Type AB responds to anything A-like or B-like as "self," so it manufactures no opposing antibodies.

Type AB presents a multifaceted, and sometimes perplexing, blood type identity. It is the first blood type to adopt an amalgamation of immune characteristics, some of which make them stronger, and some of which are in conflict. Perhaps Type AB presents the perfect metaphor for modern life: complex and unsettled.

The Blending Grounds

BLOOD TYPE, geography, and race are woven together to form our human identity. We may have cultural differences, but when you look at blood type, you see how superficial they are. Your blood

type is older than your race and more fundamental than your eth-
nicity. The blood types were not a hit-or-miss act of random genetic activity. Each new blood type was an evolutionary response
to a series of cataclysmic chain reactions, spread over eons of environmental upheaval and change.

Although the early racial changes seem to have occurred in a
world that was composed almost exclusively of Type O blood, the
racial diversifications—coupled with dietary, environmental, and
geographical adaptations—were part of the evolutionary engine
that ultimately produced the other blood types.

Some anthropologists believe that classifying humans into
races invites oversimplification. Blood type is a far more important determinant of individuality and similarity than is race. For
example, an African and Caucasian of Type A blood could exchange blood or organs and have many of the same aptitudes, digestive functions, and immunological structures—characteristics
they would not share with a member of their own race who was
Blood Type B.

Racial distinctions based on skin colors, ethnic practices, geographical homelands, or cultural roots are not a valid way to distinguish peoples. Members of the human race have a lot more in
common with one another than we may have ever suspected. We
are all potentially brothers and sisters. In blood.

Today, as we look back on this remarkable evolutionary revolution, it is clear that our ancestors had unique biological blueprints
that complemented their environments. It is this lesson we bring
with us into our current understanding of blood types, for the genetic characteristics of our ancestors live in our blood today.

- TYPE O: The oldest and most basic blood type, the survivor at the top of the food chain, with a strong and ornery
  immune system willing to and capable of destroying
  anyone, friend or foe.
- TYPE A: The first immigrants, forced by the necessity of
  migration to adapt to a more agrarian diet and lifestyle . . .

with a more cooperative personality to get along in crowded communities.

- TYPE B: The assimilator, adapting to new climates and the mingling of populations; representing nature's quest for a more balanced force between the tensions of the mind and the demands of the immune system.

- TYPE AB: The delicate offspring of a rare merger between the tolerant Type A and the formerly barbaric but more balanced Type B.

Our ancestors left each of us a special legacy, imprinted in our blood types. This legacy exists permanently in the nucleus of each cell. It is here that the anthropology and science of our blood meet.

Blood Code:

The Blueprint
of Blood Type

BLOOD IS A FORCE OF NATURE, THE ÉLAN VITAL THAT has sustained us since time immemorial. A single drop of blood, too small to see with the naked eye, contains the entire genetic code of a human being. The DNA blueprint is intact and replicated within us endlessly—through our blood.

Our blood also contains eons of genetic memory—bits and pieces of specific programming, passed on from our ancestors in codes we are still attempting to comprehend. One such code rests within our blood type. Perhaps it is the most important code we can decipher in our attempt to unravel the mysteries of blood and its vital role in our existence.

To the naked eye, blood is a homogeneous red liquid. But under the microscope, blood shows itself to be composed of many different elements. The abundant red blood cells contain a special type of iron that our bodies use to carry oxygen and create the blood's characteristic rust color. White blood cells, far less numerous than red, cruise our bloodstreams like ever-vigilant troops, protecting us against infection.

This complex, living fluid also contains proteins that deliver nutrients to the tissues, platelets that help it clot, and plasma that contains the guardians of our immune system.

The Importance of Blood Type

YOU MAY BE UNAWARE of your own blood type unless you've donated blood or needed a transfusion. Most people think of blood type as an inert factor, something that comes into play only when there is a hospital emergency. But now that you have heard the dramatic story of the evolution of blood type, you are beginning to understand that blood type has always been the driving force behind human survival, changing and adapting to new conditions, environments, and food supplies.

Why is our blood type so powerful? What is the essential role it plays in our survival—not just thousands of years in the past, but today?

Your blood type is the key to your body's entire immune system. It controls the influence of viruses, bacteria, infections, chemicals, stress, and the entire assortment of invaders and conditions that might compromise your immune system.

The word *immune* comes from the Latin *immunis*, which denoted a city in the Roman Empire that was not required to pay taxes. (If only your blood type could give you that kind of immunity!) The immune system works to define "self" and destroy "non-self." This is a critical function, for without it your immune system could attack your own tissues by mistake or allow a dangerous organism access to vital areas of your body. In spite of all its complexity, the immune system boils down to two basic functions: recognizing "us" and killing "them." In this respect your body is like a large invitation-only party. If the prospective guest supplies the correct invitation, the security guards allow him to enter and enjoy himself. If an invitation is lacking or forged, the guest is forcibly removed.

Enter the Blood Type

NATURE HAS ENDOWED our immune system with very sophisticated methods to determine if a substance in the body is foreign or not. One method involves chemical markers called *antigens*, which are found on the cells of our bodies. Every life-form, from the simplest virus to humans themselves, has unique antigens that form a part of its chemical fingerprint. One of the most powerful antigens in the human body is the one that determines your blood type. The different blood type antigens are so sensitive that when they are operating effectively, they are the immune system's greatest security system. When your immune system sizes up a suspicious character (i.e., a foreign antigen from bacteria) one of the first things it looks for is your blood type antigen to tell it whether the intruder is friend or foe.

Each blood type possesses a different antigen with its own special chemical structure. Your blood type is named for the blood type antigen you possess on your red blood cells.

IF YOU ARE	YOU HAVE THIS ANTIGEN(S) ON YOUR CELLS
BLOOD TYPE A	A
BLOOD TYPE B	B
BLOOD TYPE AB	A and B
BLOOD TYPE O	NO ANTIGENS

Visualize the chemical structure of blood types as antennae of sorts, projecting outward from the surface of our cells into deep space. These antennae are made from long chains of a repeating sugar called fucose, which by itself forms the simplest of the blood types, Blood Type O. The early discoverers of blood type called it "O" as a way to make us think of "zero" or "no real antigen." This antenna also serves as the base for the other Blood Types, A, B, and AB.

- BLOOD TYPE A is formed when the O antigen, or fucose, plus another sugar called N-acetyl-galactosamine, is added. So fucose plus N-acetyl-galactosamine equals Blood Type A.
- BLOOD TYPE B is also based on the O antigen, or fucose, but has a different sugar, named D-galactosamine, added on. So fucose plus D-galactosamine equals Blood Type B.
- BLOOD TYPE AB is based on the O antigen, fucose, plus the two sugars, N-acetyl-galactosamine and D-galacto-samine. So fucose plus N-acetyl-galactosamine plus D-galactosamine equals Blood Type AB.

The Four Blood Types And Their Antigens

The four blood types and their antigens. Type O is the stalk, fucose; Type A is fucose plus the sugar N-acetyl-galactosamine; Type B is fucose plus the sugar D-galactosamine; Type AB is fucose plus the A-sugar and the B-sugar.

At this point you may be wondering about other blood type identifiers, such as positive and negative, or secretor/non-secretor. Usually, when people tell their blood types they say, "I'm A positive." Or "I'm O negative." These variations, or subgroups, within blood types play relatively insignificant roles. More than 90 percent of all the factors associated with your blood type are related to your primary type—O, A, B, or AB. (See Appendix D for details on the meaning of the subgroups.) We will concentrate on your blood type itself.

Antigens Create Antibodies (Immune System Smart Bombs)

WHEN YOUR BLOOD TYPE ANTIGEN SENSES that a foreign antigen has entered the system, the first thing it does is create antibodies to that antigen. These antibodies, specialized chemicals manufactured by the cells of the immune system, are designed to attach to and tag the foreign antigen for destruction.

Antibodies are the cellular equivalent of the military's smart bomb. The cells of our immune system manufacture countless varieties of antibodies, and each is specifically designed to identify and attach to one particular foreign antigen. A continual battle wages between the immune system and intruders that try to change or mutate their antigens into some new form the body will not recognize. The immune system responds to this challenge with an ever-increasing inventory of antibodies.

When an antibody encounters the antigen of a microbial interloper, a reaction called agglutination (literally, gluing) occurs. The antibody attaches to the viral antigen and makes it very sticky. When cells, viruses, parasites and bacteria are agglutinated, they stick together and clump up, which makes the job of their disposal all the easier. As microbes must rely on their slippery powers of evasion, this is a very powerful defense mechanism. It is rather like handcuffing criminals together; they become far less dangerous than when they are allowed to move around freely. Sweeping the system of odd cells, viruses, parasites, and bacteria, the antibodies herd the undesirables together for easy identification and disposal.

The system of blood type antigens and antibodies has other ramifications besides detecting microbial and other invaders. Nearly one hundred years ago, Dr. Karl Landsteiner, a brilliant Austrian physician and scientist, also found that blood types produced antibodies to other blood types. His revolutionary discovery explained why some people could exchange blood, while others could not. Until Dr. Landsteiner's time, blood transfusions were a hit-or-miss affair. Sometimes they "took," and sometimes they didn't, and nobody knew why. Thanks to Dr. Landsteiner, we now know which blood types are recognized as friend by other blood types, and which are recognized as foe.

Dr. Landsteiner learned that:

- BLOOD TYPE A carried anti-B antibodies. Type B would be rejected by Type A.
- BLOOD TYPE B carried anti-A antibodies. Type A would be rejected by Type B.

Thus, Type A and Type B could not exchange blood.

- BLOOD TYPE AB carried no antibodies. The universal receiver, it would accept any other blood type! But because it carried both A and B antigens, it would be rejected by all other blood types.

Thus, Type AB could receive blood from everyone, but could give blood to no one. Except another Type AB, of course.

- BLOOD TYPE O carried anti-A and anti-B antibodies. Type A, Type B, and Type AB would be rejected.

Thus, Type O could not receive blood from anyone but another Type O. But free of A-like and B-like antigens, Type O could give blood to everyone else. Type O is the universal donor!

IF YOU ARE	YOU CARRY ANTIBODIES AGAINST
BLOOD TYPE A	BLOOD TYPE B
BLOOD TYPE B	BLOOD TYPE A
BLOOD TYPE AB	NO ANTIBODIES
BLOOD TYPE O	BLOOD TYPES A and B

The "anti-other-blood-type" antibodies are the strongest antibodies in our immune system, and their ability to clump—agglutinate—the blood cells of an opposing blood type is so powerful that it can be immediately observed on a glass slide with the unaided eye. Most of our other antibodies require some sort of stimulation (such as a vaccination or an infection) for their production. The blood type antibodies are different: they are produced automatically, often appearing at birth and reaching almost adult levels by four months of age.

But there was much more to the agglutination story. It was also found that many foods agglutinate the cells of certain blood types (in a way similar to rejection) but not others, meaning that a food which may be harmful to the cells of one blood type may be beneficial to the cells of another. Not surprisingly, many of the antigens in these foods had A-like or B-like characteristics. This discovery provided the scientific link between blood type and diet. Remarkably, however, its revolutionary implications would lie dormant, gathering dust for most of this century—until a handful of scientists, doctors, and nutritionists began to explore the connection.

Lectins: The Diet Connection

A CHEMICAL REACTION OCCURS between your blood and the foods you eat. This reaction is part of your genetic inheritance. It is amazing but true that today, in the late twentieth century, your immune and digestive systems still maintain a favoritism for foods that your blood type ancestors ate.

We know this because of a factor called lectins. Lectins, abundant and diverse proteins found in foods, have agglutinating properties that affect your blood. Lectins are a powerful way for organisms in nature to attach themselves to other organisms in nature. Lots of germs, and even our own immune systems, use this super glue to their benefit. For example, cells in our liver's bile ducts have lectins on their surfaces to help them snatch up bacteria and parasites. Bacteria and other microbes have lectins on their surfaces as well, which work rather like suction cups, so that they can attach to the slippery mucosal linings of the body. Often the lectins used by viruses or bacteria can be blood type specific, making them a stickier pest for people of that blood type.

So, too, with the lectins in food. Simply put, when you eat a food containing protein lectins that are incompatible with your blood type antigen, the lectins target an organ or bodily system (kidneys, liver, brain, stomach, etc.) and begin to agglutinate blood cells in that area.

Many food lectins have characteristics that are close enough to a certain blood type antigen to make it an "enemy" to another. For example, milk has B-like qualities; if a person with Type A blood drinks it, his system will immediately start the agglutination process in order to reject it.

Here's an example of how a lectin agglutinates in the body. Let's say a Type A person eats a plate of lima beans. The lima beans are digested in the stomach through the process of acid hydrolysis. However, the lectin protein is resistant to acid hydrolysis. It doesn't get digested, but stays intact. It may interact directly with the lining of the stomach or intestinal tract, or it may get absorbed into your bloodstream along with the digested lima bean nutrients. Different lectins target different organs and body systems.

Once the intact lectin protein settles someplace in your body, it literally has a magnetic effect on the cells in that region. It clumps the cells together and they are targeted for destruction, as if they, too, were foreign invaders. This clumping can cause irritable bowel syndrome in the intestines or cirrhosis in the liver, or block the flow of blood through the kidneys—to name just a few of the effects.

Lectins: A Dangerous Glue

YOU MAY REMEMBER the bizarre assassination of Gyorgi Markov in 1978 on a London street. Markov was killed by an unknown Soviet KGB agent while waiting for a bus. Initially, the autopsy could not pinpoint how it was done. After a thorough search, a tiny gold bead was found embedded in Markov's leg. The bead was found to be permeated with a chemical called ricin, which is a toxic lectin extracted from castor beans. Ricin is so potent an agglutinin that even an infinitesimally small amount can cause death by swiftly converting the body's red blood cells into large clots which block the arteries. Ricin kills instantaneously.

Fortunately, most lectins found in the diet are not quite so life threatening, although they can cause a variety of other problems, especially if they are specific to a particular blood type. For the most part our immune systems protect us from lectins. Ninety-five percent of the lectins we absorb from our typical diets are sloughed off by the body. But at least 5 percent of the lectins we eat are filtered into the bloodstream, where they react with and destroy red and white blood cells. The actions of lectins in the digestive tract can be even more powerful. There they often create a violent inflammation of the sensitive mucous of the intestines, and this agglutinative action may mimic food allergies. Even a minute quantity of a lectin is capable of agglutinating a huge number of cells if the particular blood type is reactive.

This is not to say that you should suddenly become fearful of every food you eat. After all, lectins are widely abundant in legumes, seafood, grains, and vegetables. It's hard to bypass them. The key is to avoid the lectins that agglutinate your particular cells—determined by blood type. For example, gluten, the most common lectin found in wheat and other grains, binds to the lining of the small intestine, causing substantial inflammation and painful irritation in some blood types—especially Type O.

Lectins vary widely, according to their source. For example, the lectin found in wheat has a different shape from the lectin found in soy, and attaches to a different combination of sugars; each of these foods is dangerous for some blood types, but beneficial for others.

Nervous tissue as a rule is very sensitive to the agglutinating effect of food lectins. This may explain why some researchers feel that allergy-avoidance diets may be of benefit in treating certain types of nervous disorders, such as hyperactivity. Russian researchers have noted that the brains of schizophrenics are more sensitive to the attachment of certain common food lectins.

Injections of lentil lectin into the knee joint cavities of non-sensitized rabbits resulted in the development of arthritis that was indistinguishable from rheumatoid arthritis. Many people with arthritis feel that avoiding the nightshade vegetables such as tomatoes, eggplant, and white potatoes seems to help their arthritis. That's not surprising, since most nightshades are very high in lectins.

Food lectins can also interact with the surface receptors of the body's white cells, programming them to multiply rapidly. These lectins are called mitogens because they cause the white cells to enter mitosis, the process of reproduction. They do not clump blood by gluing cells together; they merely attach themselves to things, like fleas on a dog. Occasionally an emergency room

Blood Type–Specific Food Lectins

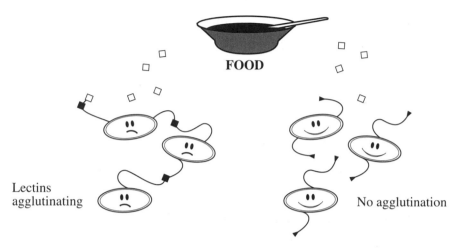

Since each blood type antigen possesses a unique shape, many lectins interact with one specific blood type because they fit the shape of that particular blood type. In the example above, food lectins from a steaming plate of lima beans interact and agglutinate Type A cells (on the left) because they fit the shape of the A antigen. The antigen for Type B blood (on the right), a different sugar molecule with a different shape, is not affected. Conversely, a food lectin (such as buckwheat) that can specifically attach to and agglutinate cells of Blood Type B would not fit Type A blood.

physician will be faced with a very ill but otherwise apparently normal child who has an extraordinarily high white blood cell count. Although pediatric leukemia is usually the first thing to come to mind, the astute physician will ask the parent, "Was your child playing in the yard?" If the answer is yes, "Was he eating any weeds or putting plants in his mouth?" Often it will turn out that the child was eating the leaves or shoots of the pokeweed plant, which contains a lectin with the potent ability to stimulate white cell production.

How to Detect
Your Harmful Lectins

I OFTEN have the experience of hearing patients insist that they are following the Blood Type Diet to the letter and staying away from all the lectins targeted for his or her blood type—but I know differently. When I challenge their assurance, usually they will drop all signs of protest and say in amazement, "How do you know?"

I know because the effects of lectins on different blood types are not just a theory. They're based on science. I've tested virtually all common foods for blood type reactions, using both clinical and laboratory methods. I can purchase isolated lectins from foods such as peanuts, lentils, meat, or wheat from chemical laboratories, and the results are visible under the microscope: I can see them agglutinating cells in the affected blood type.

There is also a more direct scientific barometer that can be used to measure the presence of lectins in your system. The barometer is a simple urine test called the Indican Scale. The Indican Scale measures a factor called bowel putrefaction. When the liver and intestines don't properly metabolize proteins, they produce toxic by-products called indols. The level of these toxic by-products is shown on the Indican Scale.

If you avoid foods containing toxic lectin proteins or foods that are difficult for your particular blood type to digest, your Indican Scale will be low.

If, on the other hand, you regularly consume foods that are high in lectins or difficult to digest, your Indican Scale will be high—meaning that you have a high carcinogenity of substances in your body.

My patients with high Indican Scale results often protest that they usually follow the diet, easing up only occasionally. They can't believe that their Indican Scale numbers are so high.

Here's the reason: the Indican Scale shows that a carcinogen entering your system is magnified to ninety times the effect of someone for whom it is not toxic. For example, if a Type A eats a processed or cured food, such as bologna, the nitrites are magnified ninety times in the negative impact they have because Type As are particularly susceptible to stomach cancer and the toxic effects of nitrites.

The average person comes into my office with a 2½ on the scale—more than enough toxicity to indicate a problem. The good news is, after only two weeks of faithfully following the Blood Type Diet, that person's Indican Scale number will drop to 1 or even 0.

This may be the first time you've ever heard of the Indican Scale, but it has been widely used in conventional medicine for the last fifty years, and all commercial laboratories perform it. Ironically, only a year ago, several major laboratory groups discontinued its use because not enough people were requesting it. I am certain that as people begin to better understand the blood type–lectin association, the Indican Scale will be revived. Meanwhile, ask your medical doctor or naturopath to perform the test.

The Indican Test

STEP 1:
Mix urine with hydrochloric acid and iron; the result will be a smoking reaction.

STEP 2:
Let the mixture sit for two minutes, then add three drops of chlorofrom. There will be more smoke–clear to dark blue in color.

STEP 3:
Measure color on the Indican Scale.

 0-2   good
 2 1/2 problems
 3-4   danger

A Blood Type Lesson: The Rabbi's Story

OVER THE YEARS, I have witnessed many transformations as a result of the Blood Type Diet. But few so moved and inspired me as my experience with a wise, elderly Brooklyn rabbi.

In early 1990, I received an urgent phone call from a New York City doctor who respected my work. He asked if I could come to see one of his patients, a renowned Hasidic rabbi who was bedridden.

"Rabbi Jacob is a very special man," he told me.

"It should be quite an experience for you—and, I hope, for him, too." He went on to tell me that the rabbi, seventy-three, had a long history of diabetes, which was poorly controlled by injectable insulin therapy. A massive stroke had left him partially paralyzed.

When I arrived to see him in his Brooklyn home, I found that Rabbi Jacob was, indeed, an impressive man who gave off an air of deep spiritual understanding and quiet compassion. Obviously once tall and strongly formed, now the rabbi lay withered and exhausted in his bed, his luxuriant white beard almost falling to his chest. In spite of his medical condition, his eyes were clear, kind, and filled with life. His main interest was getting out of bed so he could go on about his work. But I could see he was in terrible pain. Even before the stroke, he told me, his legs had been giving him problems. Poor circulation had caused swelling and inflammation in both legs and caused him to experience excruciating jolts of "pins and needles" when he tried to walk. Now his left leg was not responding to his bidding.

I wasn't surprised to learn that Rabbi Jacob was Blood Type B. Although this blood type is relatively uncommon in America, it is very common among Hasidic Jews, the majority of whom emigrated from eastern Europe.

I realized that in order to help the rabbi, I must first learn something about the way he lived and the foods he ate. Food is intimately bound to ritual in Jewish tradition.

I sat down with Rabbi Jacob's wife and daughter, both of whom were unfamiliar with naturopathic treatments. But they wanted to help the rabbi, and they were eager to learn.

"Tell me about the rabbi's diet," I said.

"He usually eats the same foods every day," his daughter told me. Those foods consisted of boiled chicken; cholent, a type of bean paste; and kasha, a buckwheat preparation. Chicken, beans, buckwheat with bow-tie noodles—these are very normal foods.

"So, how is kasha made?" I innocently asked. There was a quick conversation back and forth between mother and daughter in Yiddish, punctuated with lovely smiles at me, and gales of laughter.

"Well," said the daughter in perfect New York English, "first you cook up the kasha—the buckwheat—then you stir it in with the bow ties. Then you serve it, say blessings, and eat."

"Do you season the kasha at all?" I again innocently asked. Another outbreak of Yiddish. Then the rabbi's daughter began.

"Kasha, Doctor, well . . . you take all the fat you pulled off the chicken while you were koshering it; you put it in a heavy saucepan with just a *bissel* [tiny bit of] chopped onion, and you cook it down. You render off the fat as it cooks down, and you've got beautiful pure chicken fat. We give it to the little ones on a piece of fresh challah bread with some salt. It's so delicious you could die!"

Yes, yes, you could, I thought darkly.

"Anyway," the rabbi's daughter continued, "you take some of the *gribbenes*, which is what's left when you cook the fat away. It's all nice and dark and crispy with the caramelized onions, and you put this on the side along with the kasha for a little treat. It tastes better than potato chips. The rabbi loves it! The chicken fat you've rendered you mix into the kasha and noodles. Oh, it's just delicious. Delicious!"

I learned that these are very common Hasidic dishes, and they made up the family's typical Sabbath meal. But it was more than just a weekly ritual for the rabbi. A pious man who spent most of his time in prayer, the rabbi thought little of food and simply ate the same meal twice daily, day after day.

Although part of a centuries-old tradition, the rabbi's diet was not a good choice for people with Type B blood. The lectins in foods such as chicken, buckwheat, beans, and corn (not to mention the *gribbenes!*) were causing the cells of his blood to agglutinate, and that was probably a major factor in his stroke. These particular lectins can also block the effects of insulin, which explains why Rabbi Jacob's diabetes became increasingly difficult to control.

I understood that Orthodox Jews obeyed the laws of kashruth—kosher—ancient dietary principles first laid out in the Old Testament of the Bible. According to these dietary laws, a number of foods are forbidden, and dairy and meat are never eaten at the same meal. In fact, there are separate pots, pans, dishes, and cutlery for dairy and meat in kosher homes. And separate sinks to wash all of these things, as well.

So I approached the matter of dietary changes carefully with the two women, not wanting to disrupt the ritual and religious associations that meant so much. I was also careful not to suggest foods that I knew to be considered unclean in their tradition.

Fortunately, there were allowable substitutes. I asked Rabbi Jacob's wife to vary the family diet, restricting the rabbi's typical dishes to once a week for the actual Sabbath meal. For his other meals I asked her to prepare lamb, fish, or turkey instead of chicken; rice or millet instead of kasha; and to vary the beans used to prepare the cholent. Finally, I prescribed several vitamin and herbal combinations to speed his recovery.

Over the next year, the rabbi made wonderful progress. Within eight weeks he was walking and doing moderate exercise, which greatly helped improve his circulation. He showed remarkable vigor for a man of his age, and shook off the effects of his stroke. At six months he was switched from injectable to oral insulin therapy—a remarkable achievement considering he had been on injectable insulin for many years. There have been no further episodes of stroke, and Rabbi Jacob's diabetes is finally under control.

Treating the rabbi gave me a new appreciation for just how ancient and fundamental the wisdom of the blood types is. It also illustrated that foods chosen for religious or cultural reasons may not always be the healthiest for a person in that culture! A five- or six-thousand-year-old tradition may appear time-honored and ancient, but many of the characteristics of our blood types are thousands of years older.

As you study your Blood Type Diet, take a lesson from the rabbi. The Blood Type Diets are not an attempt to superimpose a rigid formula on your diet, or to rob you of the foods that are important to your culture. Rather, they are a way to fully support your most basic identity—to lead you back to the essential truths that live in every cell of your body and link you to your historical, evolutionary ancestry.

THREE

The Blood Type Solution:

A Road Map

*Y*OUR BLOOD TYPE PLAN LETS YOU ZERO IN ON THE health and nutrition information that corresponds to your exact biological profile. Armed with this new information, you can now make choices about your diet, exercise regimen, and general health that are based on the dynamic natural forces within your own body. The next four sections supply highly specific diet, supplement, and exercise plans for each of the blood types. These sections are followed, in Part III, by a thorough breakdown of every common health condition and disease, with your particular blood type susceptibilities and remedies. If you follow your Blood Type Plan carefully, you can:

- Avoid many common viruses and infections.
- Lose weight, as your body rids itself of toxins and fats.
- Fight back against life-threatening diseases such as cancer, cardiovascular disease, diabetes, and liver failure.
- Avoid many of the factors that cause rapid cell deterioration, thus slowing down the aging process.

The Blood Type Plan is not a panacea. But it is a way to re-store the natural protective functions of your immune system, re-set your metabolic clock, and clear your blood of dangerous agglutinating lectins. It is literally the best thing you can do to halt the rapid cell deterioration that produces symptoms of aging. And if you have medical problems, this plan can make a critical difference. Depending on the severity of the condition and on the level of compliance with the plan, every person will realize some benefits. That has been my experience, and the experience of my colleagues who use this system with thousands of patients. It makes perfect scientific sense.

In this chapter I will introduce the elements you will find in your Blood Type Plan. They include:

- The Blood Type Diet
- Meal Planning
- The Weight-Loss Factor
- The Supplement Advisory
- The Stress/Exercise Profile
- The Personality Question

After you read this chapter and review your Blood Type Plan, I suggest you read Part III to get a fuller picture of the specific medical implications your plan has for you.

The Blood Type Diet

Your blood type diet is the restoration of your natural genetic rhythm. The groundwork for the Blood Type Diets was prepared for us many thousands of years ago. Perhaps if we had continued to follow the inherent, instinctual messages of our biological na-tures, our current condition would be very different. However, hu-man diversity and the sweeping forces of technology intervened.

As we know, most, if not all, early humans were Type O hunters and gatherers who fed on animals, insects, berries, roots, and leaves. The range of dietary choices was extended when humans learned how to raise animals for their own use and how to cultivate crops. But it was not necessarily a smooth and orderly process because not every society adapted well to this change. In many of the early Type O societies, such as the Missouri Valley Indians, the change from a meat-eating diet to an agrarian diet was accompanied by changes in skull formation and the appearance for the first time of dental cavities. Their systems were simply not suited to the newly introduced foods.

Even so, for a long period of time, the traditional agrarian diet provided ample nutrients to avoid malnutrition and support large populations. This changed as advances in agricultural and food-processing techniques began to alter foodstuffs even further and remove them more and more from their natural state. For example, the refining of rice with new milling techniques in twentieth-century Asia caused a scourge of beriberi, a thiamine-deficiency disease, which resulted in millions of deaths.

A more current example is the change from breast feeding to bottle feeding in developing Third World countries. This change to highly refined, processed infant formula has been responsible for a great deal of malnutrition, diarrhea, and a lowering of the natural immune factors passed on through mother's milk.

Today, it is well accepted that nutrition—or the foods we eat—has a direct impact on the state of our health and general well-being. But confusing, and often conflicting, information about nutrition has created a virtual minefield for health-conscious consumers.

How are we to choose which recommendations to follow, and which diet is the right diet? The truth is, we can no more choose the right diet than we can choose our hair color or gender. It was already chosen for us many thousands of years ago.

I believe that much of the confusion is the result of a cavalier "one diet fits all" premise. Although we have seen with our own eyes that certain people respond very well to particular diets while others do not, we have never made a commitment—in science or nutrition—to study the specialized characteristics of populations or individuals that might explain the variety of responses to any given diet. We've been so busy looking at the characteristics of food that we have failed to examine the characteristics of people.

Your blood type diet works because you are able to follow a clear, logical, scientifically researched and certified dietary blueprint based on your cellular profile.

Each of the blood type diets includes sixteen food groups:

- Meats and poultry
- Seafood
- Dairy and eggs
- Oils and fats
- Nuts and seeds
- Beans and legumes
- Cereals
- Breads and muffins
- Grains and pasta
- Vegetables
- Fruit
- Juices and fluids
- Spices
- Condiments
- Herbal teas
- Miscellaneous beverages

Each of these groups divides foods into three categories: HIGHLY BENEFICIAL, NEUTRAL, and AVOID. Think of the categories this way:

- HIGHLY BENEFICIAL is a food that acts like a MEDICINE.
- NEUTRAL is a food that acts like a FOOD.
- AVOID is a food that acts like a POISON.

There are a wide variety of foods in each diet, so don't worry about limitations. When possible, show preference for the highly beneficial foods over the neutral foods, but feel free to enjoy the neutral foods that suit you; they won't harm you from the standpoint of lectins, and they contain nutrients that are necessary for a balanced diet.

At the top of each food category, you will see a chart that looks something like this:

BLOOD TYPE O		WEEKLY ■ IF YOUR ANCESTRY IS		
Food	*Portion*	*African*	*Caucasian*	*Asian*
ALL SEAFOOD	4–6 oz.	1–4x	3–5x	4–6x

The portion suggestions according to ancestry are not meant as firm rules. My purpose here is to present a way to fine-tune your diet even more, according to what we know about the particulars of your ancestry. Although people of different races and cultures may share a blood type, they don't always have the same frequency of the gene. For example, a Type A person may be AA, meaning both parents were As, or AO, meaning one parent was O. Overall, people of Caucasian ancestry tend to have more AA genes; people of African ancestry tend to have more OO genes; and people of Asian ancestry tend to have more BB or AA genes. That is one reason why many people of African descent are lactose intolerant, even if they are Type B (a blood type that benefits from dairy foods).

There are also geographic and cultural variations. For example, people of Asian ancestry are not traditionally exposed to dairy products, so Type Bs of Asian descent may need to incorporate them more slowly into their diets as they adjust their systems to them.

These refinements also take into account typical differences in the size and weight of various peoples. Use the refinements if you think they're helpful; ignore them if you find that they're not. In any case, try to formulate your own plan for portion sizes.

At the back of each Blood Type Diet are three sample menus and several recipes to give you an idea of how you might incorporate the diet into your life.

The Weight-Loss Factor

BEING OVERWEIGHT was anathema to our ancient ancestors, whose bodies were machines that consumed and expended the fuel they needed. Today, obesity has become one of the biggest health problems in most industrialized societies. For this reason, losing weight has become an obsession, and naturally many of my patients are interested in the weight-loss aspects of the Blood Type Diet. I always tell them that this diet was not specifically designed for weight loss; it was designed for optimum performance. Having said that, I add that weight loss is one of the natural side effects of the body's restoration. Because the Blood Type Diet is tailored to the cellular composition of your body (as opposed to being a generic, one-size-fits-all recommendation), specific foods will cause weight gain or weight loss for you, even though they may have a different effect on a person of another blood type.

My patients often ask me about current diet plans that are in vogue. The latest are the high-protein diets, which have made a recent comeback. By severely limiting carbohydrates, high-protein diets force the burning of fats for energy and the production of ketones, which indicate a high rate of metabolic activity. It doesn't surprise me that the patients who tell me they have lost weight on high-protein diets are usually Type Os and Type Bs. You don't see many Type As who do well on these diets; their systems are biologically unsuited to metabolize meat as efficiently as Type Os and Type Bs. Nor do Type ABs lose weight on high-protein diets, since these diets lack the balance of A-like foods that Type ABs require.

On the other hand, the principles of a macrobiotic diet, which encourage the consumption of natural foods such as vegetables, rice, whole grains, fruits, and soy, might be best suited for Type As, providing they eat the recommended grains and legumes.

The bottom line: Anytime you see a new diet plan that claims to work the same way for everyone, be skeptical. Listen to your blood type. Appreciate your individuality.

Let me tell you about the weight-loss potential of each of the blood type diets. Actually, the greatest problem most of my patients encounter is that they lose too much weight very quickly and I have to make adjustments in their diets to slow down the rate of weight loss. Too much weight loss may seem to be the least of your problems if you've always struggled with your weight. But remember, your ultimate goal is optimum health and performance, and that means achieving a balance between your weight and your height and shape. Excessive weight loss indicates a malnourished state that will weaken your immune system—exactly what you are trying to avoid. So use these guidelines wisely.

The dynamics of weight loss are related to the changes your body makes when you follow your genetically tailored diet. There are two factors.

First, as your body makes the dramatic shift of eliminating foods that are poorly digested or toxic, the first thing it does is try to flush out the toxins that are already there. Those toxins are deposited mainly in the fat tissue, so the process of eliminating toxins also means eliminating fat.

The second factor is the effects that specific foods have on the bodily systems that control weight. Depending on your blood type, the lectin activity of certain foods may do the following:

- Inflame the digestive tract lining.
- Interfere with the digestive process, causing bloating.
- Slow down the rate of food metabolism, so you don't efficiently burn calories for energy.
- Compromise the production of insulin.
- Upset the hormonal balance, causing water retention (edema), thyroid disorders, and other problems.

Each blood type has its own reactions to certain foods; these are outlined in your Blood Type Diet. In the first few weeks you'll need to experiment with the guidelines. I've found that many people approach their diet religiously in the beginning. They eat only the HIGHLY BENEFICIAL foods, and don't consume even NEUTRAL foods. The result is inevitably a rather unhealthy weight loss. They look gaunt and unwell because they're not getting the full range of nutrients needed for a healthy diet. A better approach is to eliminate all the foods on your AVOID list and reduce or eliminate those NEUTRAL foods that are prone to cause weight gain for your blood type. That will leave you with a balanced diet and a healthier method of weight loss.

The Role of Supplements

YOUR BLOOD TYPE PLAN also includes recommendations about vitamin, mineral, and herbal supplements that can enhance the effects of your diet. This is another area in which there is great confusion and misinformation. Popping vitamins, minerals, exotic preparations, and herbal tinctures is a popular thing to do these days. It's hard not to be seduced by the vast array of remedies overflowing the shelves of your local health food store. Promising energy, weight loss, pain relief, sexual potency, strength, longevity, and mental power—along with cures for headaches, colds, nerves, stomach pain, arthritis, chronic fatigue, heart disease, cancer, and every other ailment in the book—these tempting panaceas seem to be the answer we've all been looking for.

But as with food, nutritional supplements don't always work the same way for everyone. Every vitamin, mineral, and herbal supplement plays a specific role in your body. The miracle remedy your Type B friend raves about may be inert or even harmful for your Type A system.

It can be dangerous to self-prescribe vitamin and mineral supplements—many of which act like drugs in your body. For example, even though they are all readily available, vitamin A, vitamin D, vitamin K, and vitamin B-3 (niacin) should be administered only under the care of a physician.

However, there are many natural substances in plants, called phytochemicals, that are more effective and less damaging than vitamins and minerals. Your Blood Type Plan recommends individualized phytochemical regimens for each blood type.

You may be unfamiliar with the term *phytochemicals*. Modern science has discovered that many of these phytochemicals, once called "weeds" or "herbs," are sources of high concentrations of biologically active compounds. These compounds are widely available in other plants, but in far smaller amounts. Many phytochemicals—which I prefer to think of as food concentrates—are antioxidants, and several of them are many times more powerful than vitamins. Interestingly, these phytochemical antioxidants exhibit a remarkable degree of tissue preference, which vitamins do not enjoy. For example, the milk thistle plant *(Silybum marianum)* and the spice turmeric *(Curcuma longa)* both have an antioxidant capability hundreds of times stronger than vitamin E, and they deposit with a great degree of preference for liver tissue. These plants are very beneficial for disorders characterized by inflammation of the liver, such as hepatitis and cirrhosis.

Your specialized program of vitamins, minerals, and phytochemicals will round out the dietary aspect of your program.

The Stress/Exercise Connection

IT IS NOT ONLY the foods you eat that determine your well-being. It is also the way your body uses those nutrients for good or ill. That's where stress comes in. The concept of stress is very prominent in modern society. We often hear people remark, "I'm so stressed," or, "My problem is too much stress." Indeed, it is true that unbridled stress reactions are associated with many illnesses. Few people realize, though, that it is not the stress itself but our reaction to the stress in our environment that depletes our immune systems and leads to illness. This reaction is as old as human history. It is caused by a natural chemical response to the perception of danger. The best way to describe the stress reaction is to get a mental picture of how the body responds to stress.

Imagine this. You are man before the dawn of civilization. You lie bundled in the dark night, pressed together with your kind, sleeping. Suddenly, a huge wild animal appears in your midst. You feel its hot, rank breath on your flesh. You see it snatch your companion with its powerful claws and tear him apart with its fierce teeth. Do you grab a weapon and try to fight? Or do you turn and run for your life?

The body's response to stress has been developed and refined over thousands of years. It is a reflex, an animal instinct, our survival mechanism for dealing with life-or-death situations. When danger of any kind is sensed, we mobilize our fight-or-flight response, and we either confront what is alarming us or flee from it—mentally or physically.

Now imagine another scenario. You are in bed asleep. All is peaceful and silent. Suddenly, there is a thunderous explosion nearby. Your walls, roof, and windows shudder. You are awake now, aren't you? And how do you feel? Probably very frightened and most definitely in some kind of heart-pounding high gear.

Alarmed, your pituitary and adrenal glands flood your bloodstream with their excitant hormones. Your pulse quickens. Your lungs suck in more oxygen to fuel your muscles. Your blood sugar soars to supply a burst of energy. Digestion slows. You break into a sweat. All of these biological responses happen in an instant, triggered by stress. They prepare you—in the same way they prepared our ancient ancestors—for fight or flight.

The moment ends. The danger passes. Your body begins to change again. In the secondary, or resistance, stage of stress, your body starts to calm down and compose itself after all of the furor caused by the release of so many chemicals. The resistance stage is usually reached when whatever caused the alarm is identified and dealt with. And then, if whatever caused the initial stress is resolved, all of the reactions disappear, and everything is once again copacetic with the body's complex response system.

If whatever caused the initial stress continues, however, the body's ability to adapt to the stress becomes exhausted. It shuts down.

Unlike our ancestors, who faced intermittent acute stresses, such as the threat of predators or starvation, we live in a highly pressured, fast-paced world that imposes chronic, prolonged stress. Even though our stress response may be less acute than that of our ancestors, the fact that it is happening continuously may make the consequences even worse. Experts generally agree that the stresses of contemporary society and the resultant diseases—of the body, the mind, and the spirit—are very much a product of our industrialized culture and unnatural style of living.

The artificial pressures and stresses of a modern technological society exhaust our built-in survival mechanisms and overwhelm us. We have become socially and culturally conditioned to suppress and thwart our most natural responses. More stress hormones are being released into our blood than we can possibly use.

What is the outcome? Stress-related disorders cause 50 to 80 percent of all illnesses in modern life. We know how powerfully the mind influences the body and the body influences the mind. The entire range of these interactions is still being explored. Problems known to be exacerbated by stress and the mind-body connection are ulcers, high blood pressure, heart disease, migraine headaches, arthritis and other inflammatory diseases, asthma and other respiratory diseases, insomnia and other sleep disorders, anorexia nervosa and other eating disorders, and a variety of skin problems ranging from hives to herpes, from eczema to psoriasis. Stress is disastrous to the immune system, leaving the body open to myriad opportunistic health problems.

However, certain stresses, such as physical or creative activity, produce pleasant emotional states which the body perceives as an enjoyably heightened mental or physical experience.

Although each of us reacts to stress in a unique way, no one is immune to its effects, especially if they are prolonged and unwanted. Many of our internal reactions to stress are ancient tunes being called up and played by our bodies—the environmental stresses that shaped the evolution of the various blood types. The cataclysmic changes in locale, climate, and diet imprinted these stress patterns into the genetic memory of each blood type, and even today determine its internal response to stress.

My father has devoted the past thirty-five years to studying the stress patterns and natural energy levels of the different blood types and devising blood type–specific exercise programs that draw from the biological profiles of each. In the process, he has observed thousands of people, adults and children alike, and his empirical observations have taken on a valid shape. His findings are remarkably consistent with everything else we know about what makes each blood type function well.

The most revolutionary aspect of my father's work is the discovery that different blood types need different forms of physical activity, or exercise, to cope with their responses to stress.

Your Blood Type Plan includes a description of your own blood type stress patterns, along with the recommended course of exercise that will turn stress into a positive force. This element provides a crucial complement to your diet.

The Personality Question

WITH ALL of these fundamental connections at work, it is not surprising that people might speculate about less tangible characteristics that might be attributed to blood type—such as personality, attitudes, and behavior.

I have experienced this personally on many occasions. People often remark about the fact that I have followed in my father's footsteps to become a naturopath. "You're a chip off the old block," some will say. Or, "I guess you inherited your father's passion for healing." And sometimes, "It looks like the D'Adamos have medical genes."

Even when the observation is made partially in jest, I sense that most people truly believe that I have inherited something besides my physiological characteristics from my father—that it isn't just an accident that I am drawn to the same work that he is drawn to.

The idea that certain inherited traits, mannerisms, emotional qualities, and life preferences are buried in our genetic makeup is well accepted, although we aren't sure how to gauge this inheritance scientifically. We don't know (yet!) of any genes for personality.

Some might argue that the way we behave has more to do with nurture than with nature. But perhaps it is both.

Recently, Beverly, a longtime patient, brought her adult daughter in to see me. Beverly had told me earlier that she was young and unmarried when her daughter was born, and she gave her up for adoption. For thirty years, Beverly never knew what had become of her daughter—until the day a familiar-looking young woman appeared on her doorstep, having found her birth mother through a search organization. It turned out that Beverly's daughter was raised on the West Coast, in a very different environment from Beverly's. Yet I was astounded to watch the two of them together. They were mother and daughter in every way. They possessed exactly the same mannerisms and accents (even though Beverly was a New Yorker and her daughter was a Californian), and they seemed to share a similar sense of humor. Amazingly, Beverly's daughter had chosen the same profession as her mother. Both were human resource managers for their companies. If ever there was evidence of a genetic connection to personality, it was sitting in my office.

Of course, I realize this evidence is anecdotal, not scientific. Most of the research into this aspect of blood types is just that. Still, the connection intrigues us because it makes some sense that there might be a causal relationship between what occurs at the cellular level of our beings and our mental, physical, and emotional tendencies as expressed by our blood type.

Evolutionary changes altered the immune systems and digestive tracts of humans, resulting in the development of the blood types. But the mental and emotional response systems were also altered by evolutionary changes, and, with this alteration, very different psychological patterns and behaviors emerged.

Each blood type waged a difficult, and very distinct, battle for its existence some far time ago. The driven loner Type O would have failed miserably in the orderly, cooperative environment of Type A—a big reason for the blood type adaptation in the first place. Would it be such a surprise to find many of these primitive characteristics hidden in some deep remove of our psyches?

The belief that personality is determined by one's blood type is held in high regard in Japan. Termed *ketsu-eki-gata*, Japanese blood type analysis is serious business. Corporate managers use it to hire workers, market researchers use it to predict buying habits, and most people use it to choose friends, romantic partners, and lifetime mates. Vending machines that offer on-the-spot blood type analysis are widespread in train stations, department stores, restaurants, and other public places. There is even a highly respected organization, the ABO Society, dedicated to helping individuals and organizations make the right decisions, consistent with blood type.

The leading proponent of the blood type–personality connection is a man named Toshitaka Nomi, whose father first pioneered the theory. In 1980, Nomi and Alexander Besher wrote a book called *You Are Your Blood Type*, which has sold more than 6 million copies in Japan. It contains personality profiles and suggestions for the various blood types—right down to what you should do for a living, whom you should marry, and the dire consequences that might befall you if you should ignore this advice.

It makes for fun reading—not unlike astrology, numerology, or other methods of finding your place in the uncertain scheme of things. I think, however, that most of the advice in the book should be taken with a grain of salt. For instance, I don't believe that a soul mate or a romantic partner should be chosen by blood type. I am Type A and I am deeply in love with my wife, Martha, who is Type O. I would hate to think that we might have been kept forever apart because of some psychic incompatibility in our blood types. We do just fine, even though mealtimes can be a little chaotic.

Furthermore, as with all attempts to label people, this one has ominous undertones. Once you say, "Type A is this," or "Type B is that," the unavoidable next step is to say, "Type B is superior," or "Only a Type O can be president." Caste systems develop. A variation of this happens every day in Japan—for example, when a company advertises that it is looking for Type Bs to fill middle management positions.

So what is the value of this speculation, and why am I including it here? It's very simple. Although I think the Japanese *ketsu-eki-gata* is extreme, I can't deny that there is probably an essential truth to the theories about a relationship between our cells and our personalities.

Modern scientists and doctors have clearly acknowledged the existence of a biological mind-body connection, and we've already demonstrated the relationship between your blood type and your response to stress earlier in this chapter. The idea that your blood type may relate to your personality is not really so strange. Indeed, if you look at each of the blood types, you can see a distinct personality emerging—the inheritance of our ancestral strengths. Perhaps this is just another way for you to play to those strengths.

The characterizations and suggestions I will make about your "blood type personality" are based on the pooled impressions made from empirical observations of thousands of people over many years. Perhaps this data will provide a fuller picture of the vital force of blood type. Just don't let it become a source of limitation—rather, let it be a source of fulfillment.

By playing to your blood type's strengths, you may be able to achieve greater efficiency and accuracy in your work, and greater emotional happiness and security in your life.

There is as yet not enough hard evidence to justify any sweeping conclusions about the use of blood type to determine personality, but a world of information is waiting to be annexed and explored. A full understanding of the unique cellular blueprint of our bodies still eludes our deepest probing.

Perhaps in the next century we will finally be able to examine some master plan; a map that will show us how to get from here to there within ourselves. But perhaps not. There is so much we don't understand, so much we may never understand. But we can speculate, reflect, and consider the many possibilities. That is why we have, as a species, developed such acute intelligence.

These elements—diet, weight management, dietary supplementation, stress control, and personal qualities—form the essential elements of your individual Blood Type Plan. Refer to them often as you begin to familiarize yourself with the specific qualities of your blood type.

But before you go any further, I suggest you do one more thing: Know your blood type!

PART II

Your
Blood Type
Plan

FOUR

Blood Type

O

Plan

TYPE O: *The Hunter*

- MEAT EATER
- HARDY DIGESTIVE TRACT
- OVERACTIVE IMMUNE SYSTEM
- INTOLERANT TO DIETARY
AND ENVIRONMENTAL ADAPTATIONS
- RESPONDS BEST TO STRESS WITH
INTENSE PHYSICAL ACTIVITY
- REQUIRES AN EFFICIENT METABOLISM
TO STAY LEAN AND ENERGETIC

The Type O Diet

TYPE OS THRIVE on intense physical exercise and animal protein. The digestive tracts of all Type Os retain the memory of ancient times. The high-protein hunter-gatherer diet and the enormous physical demands placed on the systems of early Type Os probably kept most primitive humans in a mild state of ketosis—a condition in which the body's metabolism is altered. Ketosis is the result of a high-protein, high-fat diet that includes very few carbohydrates. The body metabolizes the proteins and fats into ketones, which are used in place of sugars in an attempt to keep glucose levels steady. The combination of ketosis, calorie deprivation, and constant physical activity made for a lean, mean hunting machine—the key to the survival of the human race.

Dietary recommendations today generally discourage the consumption of too much animal protein because saturated fats have been proven to be a risk factor for heart disease and cancer. Of course, most of the meat consumed today is shot through with fat and tainted by the indiscriminate use of hormones and antibiotics. "You are what you eat" can take on an ominous meaning when you're talking about the modern meat supply.

Fortunately, organic and free-range meats are becoming more widely available. The success of the Type O Diet depends on your use of lean, chemical-free meats, poultry, and fish.

Type Os don't find dairy products and grains quite as user friendly as do most of the other blood types because their digestive systems still have not adapted to them fully. After all, you don't have to chase down and kill a bowl of wheat or a glass of milk! These foods did not become staples of the human diet until much later in the course of our evolution.

The Weight-Loss Factor

YOU WILL LOSE WEIGHT INITIALLY on the Type O Diet by restricting your consumption of grains, breads, legumes, and beans. The leading factor in weight gain for Type Os is the gluten found in wheat germ and whole wheat products. It acts on your metabolism to create the exact opposite of the state of ketosis. Instead of keeping you lean and in a high-energy state, the gluten lectins inhibit your insulin metabolism, interfering with the efficient use of calories for energy. Eating gluten is like putting the wrong kind of octane in your car. Instead of fueling the engine, it clogs the works. (To a lesser extent, corn has the same effect, although it's not nearly as influential as wheat in precipitating Type O weight gain.) I have seen overweight Type Os, who had been unsuccessful with other diets, quickly lose weight solely by eliminating wheat from their diets.

Other factors contribute to weight gain in Type Os. Certain beans and legumes, especially lentils and kidney beans, contain lectins that deposit in your muscle tissues, making them more alkaline and less "charged" for physical activity. Type Os are leaner when their muscle tissues are in a state of slight metabolic acidity. In this state, you use calories more rapidly. (Before you jump to broad conclusions about other blood types, remember that each blood type has a unique set of factors. Metabolic acidity is not good for everyone.)

A third factor in Type O weight gain is related to thyroid regulation. Type Os have a tendency to have low levels of thyroid hormone. This condition, called hypothyroidism, occurs because Type Os often exhibit insufficient levels of iodine—a chemical element whose sole purpose is thyroid hormone production. The symptoms of hypothyroidism include weight gain, fluid retention, muscle loss, and fatigue.

In addition to moderating food portions and choosing leaner meats for maximum weight-control benefits, Type Os need to highlight certain foods for their beneficial effects and avoid others for their hindering effects. Here's a quick guide:

FOODS THAT ENCOURAGE WEIGHT GAIN

WHEAT GLUTEN	*interferes with insulin efficiency* *slows metabolic rate*
CORN	*interferes with insulin efficiency* *slows metabolic rate*
KIDNEY BEANS	*impair calorie utilization*
NAVY BEANS	*impair calorie utilization*
LENTILS	*inhibit proper nutrient metabolism*
CABBAGE	*inhibits thyroid hormone*
BRUSSELS SPROUTS	*inhibit thyroid hormone*
CAULIFLOWER	*inhibits thyroid hormone*
MUSTARD GREENS	*inhibit thyroid production*

FOODS THAT ENCOURAGE WEIGHT LOSS

KELP	*contains iodine* *increases thyroid hormone production*
SEAFOOD	*contains iodine* *increases thyroid hormone production*
*IODIZED SALT	*contains iodine* *increases thyroid hormone production*
LIVER	*B-vitamin source* *aids efficient metabolism*
RED MEAT	*aids efficient metabolism*
KALE, SPINACH, BROCCOLI	*aid efficient metabolism*

* It is preferable that you obtain your iodine from sources such as seafood and kelp, as sodium can contribute to high blood pressure and water retention.

INCORPORATE THESE GUIDELINES INTO THE TOTAL PICTURE OF THE TYPE O DIET, WHICH FOLLOWS.

Meats and Poultry

BLOOD TYPE O	WEEKLY ▪ IF YOUR ANCESTRY IS			
Food	*Portion**	*African*	*Caucasian*	*Asian*
LEAN RED MEATS	4–6 oz. *(men)* 2–5 oz. *(women and children)*	5–7x	4–6x	3–5x
POULTRY	4–6 oz. *(men)* 2–5 oz. *(women and children)*	1–2x	2–3x	3–4x

* The portion recommendations are merely guidelines that can help refine your diet according to ancestral propensities.

Eat lean beef, lamb, turkey, chicken, or the recommended fish as often as you wish. The more stressful your job or demanding your exercise program, the higher the grade of protein you should eat. But beware of portion sizes. Our ancestors didn't feast on sixteen-ounce steaks; meat was too precious and scarce for that. Try to consume no more than six ounces at any one meal.

Type Os can efficiently digest and metabolize meats because they tend to have high stomach-acid content. This was an essential component in the survival of early Type Os. However, you must be careful to balance your meat proteins with the appropriate vegetables and fruits to avoid over-acidification, which can cause ulcers and irritation of the stomach lining.

One note: If you are a Type O of African descent, emphasize lean red meats and game over fattier, more domestic choices such as lamb or chicken. The gene for Type O developed in Africa, and your ancestors were the original Type Os. You'll benefit by refining your protein consumption in favor of the varieties of meat that were available to your African ancestors.

Highly Beneficial

BEEF	HEART	MUTTON
BEEF, GROUND	LAMB	VEAL
BUFFALO	LIVER	VENISON

Neutral

Chicken	Partridge	Turkey
Cornish hens	Pheasant	Quail
Duck	Rabbit	

Avoid

Bacon	Ham
Goose	Pork

Seafood

BLOOD TYPE O		WEEKLY ▪ IF YOUR ANCESTRY IS		
Food	*Portion*	*African*	*Caucasian*	*Asian*
ALL SEAFOOD	4–6 OZ.	1–4X	3–5X	4–6X

Seafood, the second most concentrated animal protein, is best suited for Type Os of Asian and Eurasian descent, since seafood was a staple of your coastal ancestors' diet.

Richly oiled cold-water fish, such as cod, herring, and mackerel, are excellent for Type Os. Certain blood clotting factors evolved as humans adapted to environmental changes, and were not inherent to the blood of early Type Os. For this reason, Type Os often have "thin" blood, which resists clotting. Even though fish oils tend to have a blood-thinning effect, they are very good for Type Os. I suspect that this is because the way their blood type genes influence their blood "thickness" (through clotting factors) is different from the way fish oils influence blood viscosity (through the adhesion of platelets). Fish oils can also be very effective in the treatment of inflammatory bowel disease, such as colitis or Crohn's disease, to which Type Os are susceptible. Many seafoods are also excellent sources of iodine, which regulates the thyroid function. Type Os typically have unstable thyroid functions, which cause metabolic problems and weight gain.

Make seafood a major component of the Type O diet.

Highly Beneficial

BLUEFISH	RAINBOW	STRIPED BASS
COD	TROUT	STURGEON
HAKE	RED SNAPPER	SWORDFISH
HALIBUT	SALMON	TILEFISH
HERRING	SARDINE	WHITE PERCH
MACKEREL	SHAD	WHITEFISH
PIKE	SNAPPER	YELLOW PERCH
	SOLE	YELLOWTAIL

Neutral

Abalone	Gray sole	Scallop
Albacore (Tuna)	Grouper	Sea bass
Anchovy	Haddock	Sea trout
Beluga	Lobster	Shark
Bluegill bass	Mahimahi	Shrimp
Carp	Monkfish	Silver perch
Clam	Mussels	Smelt
Crab	Ocean perch	Snail
Crayfish	Oysters	Squid (calamari)
Eel	Pickerel	Turtle
Flounder	Porgy	Weakfish
Frog	Sailfish	

Avoid

Barracuda	Herring (pickled)
Catfish	Lox (smoked salmon)
Caviar	Octopus
Conch	

Dairy and Eggs

BLOOD TYPE O	WEEKLY ■ IF YOUR ANCESTRY IS			
Food	*Portion*	*African*	*Caucasian*	*Asian*
EGGS	I EGG	0	3–4X	5X
CHEESES	2 OUNCES	0	0–3X	0–3X
YOGURT	4–6 OUNCES	0	0–3X	0–3X
MILK	4–6 OUNCES	0	0–IX	0–2X

Type Os should severely restrict their use of dairy products. Their system is ill designed for their proper metabolism, and there are no highly beneficial foods in this group.

If you are a Type O of African ancestry, you should eliminate dairy foods and eggs altogether. They tend to be even more difficult for you to digest; indeed, many African-Americans are lactose intolerant. Soy milk and soy cheese are excellent, high-protein alternatives.

Food allergies are not digestive problems. They are immune system reactions to certain foods. Your immune system literally creates an antibody that fights the intrusion of the food into your system. Food intolerances, on the other hand, are digestive reactions that can occur for many reasons, including cultural conditioning, psychological associations, poor-quality food, additives, or just some undefinable quirk in your own system. It makes sense that African-Americans might be lactose intolerant, since their hunter-gatherer African ancestors had no lactose in their diets.

Other Type Os may eat four or five eggs a week and small amounts of dairy, but it is generally a poor protein source for your blood type. Be sure, however, to take a daily calcium supplement, especially if you are a woman, since dairy foods are the best natural source of absorbable calcium.

Neutral

Butter	Mozzarella
Farmer	Soy cheese*
Feta	Soy milk*
Goat cheese	

Good dairy alternatives

Avoid

American cheese	Edam	Parmesan
Blue cheese	Emmenthal	Provolone
Brie	Goat milk	Neufchatel
Buttermilk	Gouda	Ricotta
Camembert	Gruyère	Skim or 2% milk
Casein	Ice cream	String cheese
Cheddar	Jarlsburg	Swiss
Colby	Kefir	Whey
Cottage	Monterey jack	Whole milk
Cream cheese	Munster	Yogurt, all varieties

Oils and Fats

BLOOD TYPE O	WEEKLY ▪ IF YOUR ANCESTRY IS			
Food	*Portion*	*African*	*Caucasian*	*Asian*
OILS	TABLESPOON	1–5x	4–8x	3–7x

Type Os respond well to oils. They can be an important source of nutrition and an aid to elimination. You will increase their value in your system if you limit your use to the monounsaturated variety, such as olive oil and flaxseed oil. These oils have positive effects on the heart and arteries, and may even help reduce blood cholesterol.

Highly Beneficial

LINSEED (FLAXSEED) OIL
OLIVE OIL

Neutral

Canola oil
Cod liver oil
Sesame oil

Avoid

Corn oil   Peanut oil
Cottonseed oil   Safflower oil

Nuts and Seeds

BLOOD TYPE O		WEEKLY ■ IF YOUR ANCESTRY IS		
Food	*Portion*	*African*	*Caucasian*	*Asian*
NUTS AND SEEDS	6–8 NUTS	2–5X	3–4X	2–3X
NUT BUTTERS	TABLESPOON	3–4X	3–7X	2–4X

Type Os can find a good source of supplemental vegetable protein from some varieties of nuts and seeds. However, these foods should in no way take the place of high-protein meats. You certainly don't need them in your diet, and should be very selective in their use, as they are high in fat. Certainly you should avoid them if you're trying to lose weight.

Since nuts can sometimes cause digestive problems, be sure to chew them thoroughly, or use nut butters, which are easier to digest, especially if you have the colon problems that are more frequently experienced by Type Os.

Highly Beneficial

PUMPKIN SEEDS
WALNUTS

Neutral

Almonds	Macadamia	Sesame seeds
Almond butter	Pecans	Sunflower butter
Chestnuts	Pignola (Pine)	Sunflower seeds
Filbert	Sesame butter	
Hickory	(tahini)	

Avoid

Brazil	Peanut butter
Cashew	Pistachios
Litchi	Poppy seeds
Peanuts	

Beans and Legumes

BLOOD TYPE O		WEEKLY ▪ IF YOUR ANCESTRY IS		
Food	*Portion*	*African*	*Caucasian*	*Asian*
ALL RECOMMENDED BEANS AND LEGUMES	1 CUP, DRY	1–2X	1–2X	2–6X

Type Os don't utilize beans particularly well, although those of Asian ancestry do a bit better because they are culturally acclimated to them. In general, beans inhibit the metabolism of other more important nutrients, such as those found in meat. They also tend to make muscle tissue slightly less acidic, and Type Os usually perform better when muscle tissues are somewhat more acidic. This is not to be confused with the acid/alkaline reaction that occurs in your stomach. In that case, the few highly beneficial beans are exceptions. They actually promote the strengthening of the digestive tract and promote healing of ulcerations—a Type O problem because of the high levels of stomach acid. Even so, eat beans in moderation, as an occasional side dish.

Highly Beneficial

BEANS, ADUKE	BEANS, PINTO
BEANS, AZUKI	PEAS, BLACK-EYED

Neutral

Beans, black	Beans, jicama	Beans, string
Beans, broad	Beans, lima	Beans, white
Beans, cannellini	Beans, northern	Peas, green
Beans, fava	Beans, red	Peas, pods
Beans, garbanzo	Beans, red soy	
Beans, green	Beans, snap	

Avoid

Beans, copper	Lentils, domestic
Beans, kidney	Lentils, green
Beans, navy	Lentils, red
Beans, tamarind	

Cereals

BLOOD TYPE O	WEEKLY ■ IF YOUR ANCESTRY IS			
Food	*Portion*	*African*	*Caucasian*	*Asian*
ALL RECOMMENDED CEREALS	I CUP, DRY	2–3X	2–3X	2–4X

Type Os do not tolerate whole wheat products at all, and you should eliminate them completely from your diet. They contain lectins that react with both your blood and your digestive tract and interfere with the proper absorption of beneficial foods. Wheat products are a primary culprit in Type O weight gain. The glutens in wheat germ interfere with Type O metabolic processes. Inefficient or sluggish metabolism causes food to convert to energy more slowly, and so store itself as fat.

Neutral

Amaranth	Kamut	Rice, puffed
Barley	Kasha	Spelt
Buckwheat	Millet, puffed	
Cream of rice	Rice bran	

Avoid

Cornflakes	Farina	Seven-grain
Cornmeal	Grape nuts	Shredded wheat
Cream of wheat	Oat bran	Wheat bran
Familia	Oatmeal	Wheat germ

Breads and Muffins

BLOOD TYPE O	DAILY ▪ IF YOUR ANCESTRY IS			
Food	*Portion*	*African*	*Caucasian*	*Asian*
BREADS, CRACKERS	I SLICE	0–4X	0–2X	0–4X
MUFFINS	I MUFFIN	0–2X	0–IX	0–IX

Obviously breads and muffins can be a source of trouble for Type Os, since most of them contain some wheat. It may be difficult at first to eliminate your morning muffin or daily sandwich; these have become staples of the American diet. Even wheat-free breads can be troublesome for Type Os if they eat them often enough; their genetic makeup is not assimilated to the consumption of grains.

Two exceptions are Essene and Ezekiel bread, which are usually found in the freezer section of your local health food store. These sprouted seed breads are assimilable to Type Os because the gluten lectins (principally found in the seed coats) are destroyed by the sprouting process. Unlike commercially produced sprouted breads, Ezekiel and Essene breads are live foods with many beneficial enzymes intact.

Highly Beneficial

ESSENE BREAD
EZEKIEL BREAD

Neutral

Brown rice bread	Millet	Rye Vita
Fin crisp	Rice cakes	Soy flour bread
Gluten-free bread	100% Rye bread	Spelt bread
Ideal Flat Bread	Rye Crisps	Wasa bread

Avoid

Bagels, wheat	Matzos, wheat	Wheat bran
Corn muffins	Multi-grain bread	muffins
Durum wheat	Oat bran muffins	Whole wheat
English muffins	Pumpernickel	bread
High-protein	Sprouted wheat	
bread	bread	

Grains and Pasta

BLOOD TYPE O		WEEKLY ▪ IF YOUR ANCESTRY IS		
Food	*Portion*	*African*	*Caucasian*	*Asian*
GRAINS	1 CUP, DRY	0–3X	0–3X	0–3X
PASTAS	1 CUP, DRY	0–3X	0–3X	0–3X

There are no grains or pastas that could be classified highly beneficial for Type Os.

Most pasta is made with semolina wheat, so you'll need to select very carefully if you want an occasional pasta dish. Pastas made from buckwheat, Jerusalem artichoke, or rice flour are better tolerated by Type Os. But these foods are not essential to your diet and should be limited in favor of more effective animal and fish foods.

Neutral

Barley flour	Quinoa	Rice, wild
Buckwheat	Rice, basmati	Rice flour
Kasha	Rice, brown	Rye flour
Pasta, artichoke	Rice, white	Spelt flour

Avoid

Bulgur wheat flour	Graham flour	Sprouted wheat flour
Couscous flour	Oat flour	White flour
Durum wheat flour	Soba noodles	Whole wheat flour
Gluten flour	Pasta, semolina	
	Pasta, spinach	

Vegetables

BLOOD TYPE O	DAILY ■ ALL ANCESTRAL TYPES
Food	*Portion*
RAW	1 CUP, PREPARED 3–5X
COOKED OR STEAMED	1 CUP, PREPARED 3–5X

There are a tremendous number of vegetables available to Type Os, and they form a critical component of your diet. You cannot, however, simply eat all vegetables indiscriminately. Several classes of vegetables cause big problems for Type Os. For example, certain vegetables from the Brassica family—cabbage, Brussels sprouts, cauliflower, and mustard greens—can inhibit the thyroid function, which is already somewhat weak in Type Os.

Leafy green vegetables rich in vitamin K, like kale, collard greens, romaine lettuce, broccoli, and spinach are very good for Type Os. This vitamin has one purpose only—to help blood clot. Type Os, as we have discussed, lack several clotting factors, and need vitamin K to assist in the process.

Alfalfa sprouts contain components that, by irritating the digestive tract, can aggravate Type O hypersensitivity problems. The molds in domestic and shiitake mushrooms, as well as fermented olives, tend to trigger allergic reactions in Type Os. All of these foods are foreign to the Type O system, which has not been designed to handle them.

The nightshade vegetables, such as eggplant and potatoes, cause arthritic conditions in Type Os because their lectins deposit in the tissue surrounding the joints.

Corn lectins affect the production of insulin, often leading to diabetes and obesity. All Type Os should avoid corn—especially if you have a weight problem or a family history of diabetes.

Tomatoes are a special case. Heavily laced with powerful lectins, called panhemaglutinans (meaning they agglutinate all blood types), tomatoes are trouble for Type A and Type B digestive tracts. However, Type Os can eat tomatoes. They become neutral in your system.

Highly Beneficial

ARTICHOKE,	COLLARD	KOHLRABI
DOMESTIC	GREENS	LEEK
ARTICHOKE,	DANDELION	LETTUCE,
JERUSALEM	ESCAROLE	ROMAINE
BEET LEAVES	GARLIC	OKRA
BROCCOLI	HORSERADISH	ONIONS, RED
CHICORY	KALE	ONIONS, SPANISH

ONIONS,
  YELLOW
PARSLEY
PARSNIPS

PEPPERS, RED
POTATOES,
  SWEET
PUMPKIN

SEAWEED
SPINACH
SWISS CHARD
TURNIPS

Neutral

Arugula
Asparagus
Bamboo shoots
Beets
Bok choy
Caraway
Carrots
Celery
Chervil
Coriander
Cucumber
Daikon
Dill
Endive
Fennel
Fiddlehead ferns
Ginger

Lettuce, Bibb
Lettuce, Boston
Lettuce, iceberg
Lettuce, mesclun
Lima beans
Mushroom,
  abalone
Mushroom, enoki
Mushroom,
  Portobello
Mushroom, tree
  oyster
Olives, green
Onions, green
Peppers, green
Peppers, jalapeno
Peppers, yellow

Radicchio
Radishes
Rappini
Rutabaga
Scallion
Shallots
Snow peas
Sprouts, mung
Sprouts, radish
Squash, all types
Tempeh
Tofu
Tomato
Water chestnut
Watercress
Yams, all types
Zucchini

Avoid

Avocado
Cabbage, Chinese
Cabbage, red
Cabbage, white
Cauliflower
Corn, white
Corn, yellow

Eggplant
Mushroom,
  domestic
Mushroom,
  shiitake
Mustard greens
Olives, black

Olives, Greek
Olives, Spanish
Potatoes, red
Potatoes, white
Sprouts, alfalfa
Sprouts, Brussels

Fruit

BLOOD TYPE O	DAILY ▪ ALL ANCESTRAL TYPES	
Food	*Portion*	
ALL RECOMMENDED FRUITS	I FRUIT OR 3–5 OZ.	3–4X

Many wonderful fruits are available on the Type O Diet. Fruits are not only an important source of fiber, vitamins, and minerals, but they can be an excellent alternative to breads and pasta for Type Os. If you eat a piece of fruit rather than a slice of bread, your system will be better served—and at the same time you'll be supporting your weight-loss goals.

It may surprise you to find some of your favorite fruits on the Avoid list, and some odd choices on the Highly Beneficial list. The reason that plums, prunes, and figs are so beneficial to your blood type is that most dark red, blue, and purple fruits tend to cause an alkaline rather than an acidic reaction in your digestive tract. The Type O digestive tract has high acidity and needs the balance of the alkaline to reduce ulcers and irritations of the stomach lining. However, just because a fruit is alkaline doesn't mean it's good for you. Melons are also alkaline, but they contain high mold counts, to which Type Os have a proven sensitivity. Most melons should be eaten in moderation, and cantaloupe and honeydew, which have the highest mold counts of all, should be avoided completely.

Oranges, tangerines, and strawberries should be avoided because of their high acid content. Grapefruit also has a high acid content, but you may eat it in moderation because it exhibits alkaline properties after digestion. Most other berries are okay, but stay away from blackberries, which contain a lectin that aggravates Type O digestion. Type Os also have an extreme sensitivity to coconut and coconut-containing products. Stay away from these, and always check food labels to be sure you're not consuming coconut oil. This oil is high in saturated fat and provides little nutritional benefit.

Highly Beneficial

FIGS, DRIED	PLUMS, DARK	PLUMS, RED
FIGS, FRESH	PLUMS, GREEN	PRUNES

Neutral

Apples	Grapes, green	Melon,
Apricots	Grapes, red	watermelon
Bananas	Guava	Nectarines
Blueberries	Kiwi	Papayas
Boysenberries	Kumquat	Peaches
Cherries	Lemons	Pears
Cranberries	Limes	Persimmons
Currants, black	Loganberries	Pineapples
Currants, red	Mangoes	Pomegranates
Dates, red	Melon, canang	Prickly pear
Elderberries	Melon, casaba	Raisins
Gooseberries	Melon, Crenshaw	Raspberries
Grapefruit	Melon, Christmas	Starfruit
Grapes, black	Melon, musk	(carambola)
Grapes, Concord	Melon, Spanish	

Avoid

Blackberries	Melon, honeydew	Rhubarb
Coconuts	Oranges	Strawberries
Melon, cantaloupe	Plantains	Tangerines

Juices and Fluids

BLOOD TYPE O	DAILY ▪ ALL ANCESTRAL TYPES	
Food	*Portion*	
ALL RECOMMENDED JUICES	8 OZ.	2–3X
WATER	8 OZ.	4–7X

Vegetable juices are preferable to fruit juices for Type Os because of their alkalinity. If you drink fruit juice, choose a low-sucrose variety. Avoid high-sugar juices such as apple juice or apple cider.

Pineapple juice can be particularly helpful in avoiding water retention and bloating, both factors which contribute to weight gain. Black cherry is also a beneficial, high-alkaline juice.

Highly Beneficial

BLACK CHERRY
PINEAPPLE
PRUNE

Neutral

Apricot	Grape	Vegetable juice
Carrot	Grapefruit	(corresponding
Celery	Papaya	with highlighted
Cranberry	Tomato water	vegetables)
Cucumber	(with lemon)	

Avoid

Apple	Cabbage
Apple cider	Orange

Spices

Your choice of spices can actually improve your digestive and immune systems. For example, kelp-based seasonings are very good for Type Os because they are rich sources of iodine, key to regulating the thyroid gland. Iodized salt is another good source of iodine, but use it sparingly.

The kelp bladder wrack tends to counter the hyperacidity of the Type O digestive tract, reducing the potential for ulcers. The abundant fucose in the kelp protects the intestinal lining of the Type O stomach, preventing ulcer-causing bacteria from adhering. Keep in mind also that kelp is highly effective as a metabolic regulator for Type Os, and is an important aid to weight loss.

Parsley is soothing to your digestive tract, as are certain warming spices, like curry and cayenne pepper. Note, however, that black and white pepper and vinegar are irritants to the Type O stomach.

Sugar products such as honey and sugar will not harm you. Nor will chocolate. But these should all be strictly limited to occasional use as condiments. Avoid corn syrup as a sweetener.

Highly Beneficial

CAROB	KELP (BLADDER	PEPPER,
CURRY	WRACK)	CAYENNE
DULSE	PARSLEY	TURMERIC

Neutral

Agar	Basil	Chives
Allspice	Bay leaf	Chocolate
Almond extract	Bergamot	Clove
Anise	Brown rice syrup	Coriander
Arrowroot	Cardamom	Cream of tartar
Barley malt	Chervil	Cumin

Dill	Pepper,	Soy sauce
Garlic	peppercorn	Spearmint
Gelatin, plain	Pepper, red	Sucanat
Honey	pepper flakes	Sugar, white
Horseradish	Peppermint	Sugar, brown
Maple syrup	Pimiento	Tamari
Marjoram	Rice syrup	Tamarind
Mint	Rosemary	Tapioca
Miso	Saffron	Tarragon
Molasses	Sage	Thyme
Mustard (dry)	Salt	Wintergreen
Paprika	Savory	

Avoid

Capers	Pepper, white
Cinnamon	Vanilla
Cornstarch	Vinegar, apple
Corn syrup	cider
Nutmeg	Vinegar, balsamic
Pepper, black	Vinegar, red wine
ground	Vinegar, white

Condiments

There are no highly beneficial condiments for Type Os. If you must have mustard or salad dressing on your foods, use them in moderation, and stick to the low-fat, low-sugar varieties.

Although Type Os can have tomatoes occasionally, avoid ketchup that also contains ingredients like vinegar.

All pickled foods are indigestible for Type Os. They severely irritate the Type O stomach lining. My recommendation is that you try to wean yourself from condiments, or replace them with healthier seasonings such as olive oil, lemon juice, and garlic.

Neutral

Apple butter	Mustard
Jam (from acceptable fruits)	Salad dressing (low-fat, from acceptable ingredients)
Jelly (from acceptable fruits)	Worcestershire sauce

Avoid

Ketchup	Pickles, kosher	Pickles, sour
Pickles, dill	Pickles, sweet	Relish
Mayonnaise		

Herbal Teas

The recommendations regarding herbal teas are based on our general understanding of what makes Type Os sick. Think of herbal teas as a way to shore up your strength against your natural weaknesses. For Type Os, the primary emphasis is on soothing the digestive and immune systems.

Herbs like peppermint, parsley, rose hip, and sarsaparilla all have that effect. On the other hand, herbs like alfalfa, aloe, burdock, and corn silk stimulate the immune system and cause blood thinning, a problem for Type Os.

Highly Beneficial

CAYENNE	HOPS	ROSE HIPS
CHICKWEED	LINDEN	SARSAPARILLA
DANDELION	MULBERRY	SLIPPERY ELM
FENUGREEK	PARSLEY	
GINGER	PEPPERMINT	

Neutral

Catnip	Dong quai	Ginseng
Chamomile	Elder	Green tea

Hawthorn	Sage	Vervain
Horehound	Skullcap	White birch
Licorice root	Spearmint	White oak bark
Mullein	Thyme	Yarrow
Raspberry leaf	Valerian	

Avoid

Alfalfa	Echinacea	Saint-John's-wort
Aloe	Gentian	Senna
Burdock	Goldenseal	Shepherd's purse
Coltsfoot	Red clover	Strawberry leaf
Corn silk	Rhubarb	Yellow dock

Miscellaneous Beverages

There are very few acceptable beverages for Type Os. You're pretty much limited to the innocuous effects of seltzer, club soda, and tea. Beer is okay in moderation, but it's not a good choice if you want to lose weight. Modest quantities of wine are allowed, but it shouldn't be a daily ritual. Green tea is allowed as an acceptable substitute for other caffeinated products, but it contains no special curative properties for Type Os. The problem that coffee poses for Type Os is in the increased levels of stomach acid it produces. Type Os have plenty of stomach acid all their own; they really don't need help. If you are a coffee drinker, perhaps you can begin to gradually cut down on the amount you consume each day. Your ultimate goal should be to eliminate drinking coffee altogether. The common withdrawal symptoms such as headache, fatigue, and irritability, won't occur if you wean yourself gradually. Green tea is a good caffeinated alternative.

Highly Beneficial

SELTZER WATER

Neutral

Beer   Wine, red
Tea, green   Wine, white

Avoid

Coffee, regular   Soda, cola   Tea, black decaf
Coffee, decaf   Soda, diet   Tea, black regular
Liquor, distilled   Soda, other

Meal Planning for Type O

Asterisk (*) indicates the recipe follows.

THE FOLLOWING sample menus and recipes will give you an idea of a typical diet beneficial to Type Os. They were developed by Dina Khader, M.S., R.D., a nutritionist who has used the blood type diets successfully with her patients.

These menus are moderate in calories and balanced for metabolic efficiency in Type Os. The average person will be able to maintain weight comfortably and even lose weight by following these suggestions. However, alternative food choices are provided if you prefer lighter fare or wish to limit your caloric intake and still eat a balanced, satisfying diet. (The alternative food is listed directly across from the food it replaces.)

Occasionally you will see an ingredient in a recipe that appears on your avoid list. If it is a very small ingredient (such as a dash of pepper), you may be able to tolerate it, depending on your condition and whether you are strictly adhering to the diet. However, the meal selections and recipes are generally designed to work very well for Type Os.

As you become more familiar with the Type O Diet recommendations, you'll be able to easily create your own menu plans and adjust favorite recipes to make them Type O–friendly.

STANDARD MENU ▪	WEIGHT-CONTROL ALTERNATIVES ▪

SAMPLE MEAL PLAN I

Breakfast

2 slices toasted Ezekiel bread with butter or organic almond butter 6 ounces vegetable juice banana green tea or herbal tea	1 slice toasted Ezekiel bread with all-natural, low-sugar jam

Lunch

*Organic Roast Beef, 6 ounces *Spinach Salad apple or pineapple slices water or seltzer	Organic Roast Beef, 2 to 4 ounces

Midafternoon snack

*1 slice Quinoa Applesauce Cake green tea or herbal tea	sliced carrot and celery sticks sliced fruits rice cakes with a drizzle of honey

Dinner

*Lamb/Asparagus Stew steamed broccoli sweet potato mixed fresh fruit—blueberries, kiwi, grapes, peaches seltzer or herbal tea (beer or wine allowed)	steamed artichoke with lemon juice avoid beer and wine

SAMPLE MEAL PLAN 2

Breakfast

2 slices Essene or Ezekiel bread with sweet butter, jam, or apple butter

2 poached eggs

6 ounces pineapple juice

green tea or herbal tea

1 slice Essene or Ezekiel bread with apple butter

1 poached egg

Lunch

chicken salad—sliced breast of chicken, mayonnaise, green grapes, walnut

1 slice rye bread or salad greens

2 plums

water or seltzer

broiled chicken breast

endive and tomato salad slivers

Midafternoon snack

pumpkin seeds and walnuts, or rice cakes with almond butter, or figs, dates, prunes

seltzer, water or herbal tea

6 oz. vegetable juice

2 Fin Crisp or rice cakes with natural, low sugar jelly

Dinner

*Arabian Baked Fish

*String Bean Salad

steamed collard greens tossed with lemon juice

green tea or herbal tea

(beer or wine allowed—but not every day)

*Baked Fish

avoid beer and wine

Sample Meal Plan 3

Breakfast

*Maple-Walnut Granola with soy milk   puffed rice with soy milk

1 poached egg

8 oz. pineapple or prune juice

green tea or herbal tea

Lunch

4–6 ounces lean ground beef patty   4-ounce ground beef patty (no bread)

2 slices Essene bread

mixed green salad—romaine, parsley, red onion carrots, cucumber

olive oil/ lemon juice dressing

water or herbal tea

Midafternoon snack

*2 Carob Chip Cookies   mixed fruit

green tea or herbal tea

Dinner

*Kifta

with grilled vegetables

brown rice with dab of butter   endive salad

herbal tea

(beer or wine allowed)   avoid beer and wine

Recipes

ORGANIC BEEF ROAST

1 beef roast (about 3 pounds)
salt, pepper, and allspice to taste
6 cloves garlic
extra-virgin olive oil
bay leaves

Remove visible fat and place roast in baking pan. Season and cut gashes, inserting cut garlic cloves, and bay leaves. Brush the meat with extra-virgin olive oil.

Place uncovered roast in 350 degree F oven for 90 minutes, or until meat is tender.

Serves 6.

QUINOA APPLESAUCE CAKE

1¾ cup quinoa flour
1 cup currants or other (allowed) dried fruit
½ cup chopped pecans
½ teaspoon baking soda
½ teaspoon aluminum-free baking powder
½ teaspoon salt
½ teaspoon ground cloves
½ cup unsalted, sweet butter or ½ cup organic canola oil
1 cup Sucanat sugar or maple sugar
1 large organic egg
2 cups unsweetened, organic applesauce

Preheat oven to 350 degrees F. Sprinkle ¼ cup of the flour over the currants and nuts and set aside. Blend the baking soda,

baking powder, salt, and cloves with the remaining quinoa
flour. Separately mix together butter or oil, sugar, and egg.
Combine all ingredients, adding the fruit and nuts at the end.
Spoon into an oiled 8 x 8-inch cake pan and bake for 40 to 45 minutes or until the cake tester inserted in the center comes out
clean.

LAMB-ASPARAGUS STEW

1 pound fresh asparagus spears
½ pound free-range lamb meat, cubed
1 medium onion, chopped
3 tablespoons organic, sweet unsalted butter
1 cup water
salt, pepper, and allspice to taste
juice of 1 lemon

Cut asparagus spears in 2-inch lengths, discarding tough portion
at bottom. Wash and drain.
Sauté meat and onions in butter until light brown. Add water,
salt, and spices. Cook until tender. Add asparagus. Simmer for
15 minutes or until tender. Add lemon juice.
Makes 2 servings.

SPINACH SALAD

2 bunches fresh spinach
1 bunch scallions, chopped
juice of 1 lemon
¼ tablespoon olive oil
salt and pepper to taste

Wash spinach well. Drain and chop. Sprinkle with salt. After a
few minutes, squeeze excess water. Add scallions, lemon
juice, oil, salt, and pepper. Serve immediately.
Makes 6 servings.

ARABIAN BAKED FISH

1 large halibut or whitefish (3 to 4 pounds)
salt and pepper to taste
¼ cup lemon juice
2 tablespoons olive oil
2 large onions, chopped and sautéed in olive oil
2 to 2½ cups tahini sauce (see below)

Preheat oven to 400 degrees F.

Wash fish and dry thoroughly. Sprinkle with salt and lemon juice. Let stand for 30 minutes. Drain fish. Brush with oil and place in baking pan. Bake for 30 minutes.

Cover with sautéed onions and tahini sauce. Sprinkle with salt and pepper. Return to oven and bake until fish is easily flaked with a fork (from 30 to 40 minutes).

Serve the fish on a platter and garnish with parsley and lemon wedges.

Makes 6 to 8 servings.

TAHINI SAUCE

1 cup organic tahini
juice of 3 lemons
2 cloves of garlic, crushed
2 to 3 teaspoons salt
¼ cup dried, organic parsley flakes or fresh parsley,
chopped finely
water

In a bowl, mix tahini with lemon juice, garlic, salt, and parsley. Add enough water to make a thick sauce.

BAKED FISH

1 large whitefish (2 or 3 pounds) or other fish
lemon juice and salt to taste
¼ cup oil
1 teaspoon cayenne
1 teaspoon cumin (optional)

Preheat oven to 350 degrees F.

Wash fish. Sprinkle with salt and lemon juice. Let stand for 30 minutes. Drain.

Coat fish with oil and spices and place in a baking pan. To prevent fish from drying, wrap with lightly oiled foil. Bake for 30 to 40 minutes, or until fish is tender and easily flaked.

Makes 4 to 5 servings.

WITH STUFFING *(OPTIONAL)*

⅓ cup pine nuts or shredded almonds
2 tablespoons sweet, unsalted butter
1 cup parsley, chopped
3 cloves garlic, crushed
salt and allspice to taste

Sauté nuts in butter until lightly brown. Add parsley and spices and sauté for one minute. Stuff raw fish with the mixture.

STRING BEAN SALAD

1 pound green string beans
juice of 1 lemon
3 tablespoons olive oil
2 cloves garlic, crushed
2 to 3 teaspoons salt

Wash tender, fresh green string beans. Remove stems and strings.
   Cut into 2-inch pieces.
Cook until tender by boiling in plenty of water. Drain. When
   cool, place in a salad bowl. Dress to taste with lemon juice,
   olive oil, garlic, and salt.
Makes 4 servings.

MAPLE-WALNUT GRANOLA

4 cups rolled oats
1 cup rice bran
1 cup sesame seeds
½ cup dried cranberries
½ cup dried currants
1 cup chopped walnuts
¼ cup organic canola oil
½ cup maple syrup
¼ cup honey
1 teaspoon vanilla extract

Preheat oven to 250 degrees F. In a large mixing bowl combine
   the oats, rice bran, seeds, dried fruit, and nuts. Add the oil and
   stir evenly.
Pour in maple syrup, honey, and vanilla and mix well until evenly
   moistened. Mixture should be crumbly and sticky. Spread
   mixture in a cookie tray and bake for 90 minutes, stirring every

15 minutes for even toasting until the mixture is golden brown and dry.

Cool well and store in airtight container.

CAROB CHIP COOKIES

⅓ cup organic canola oil
½ cup pure maple syrup
1 teaspoon vanilla extract
1 organic egg
1¾ cups oat or brown rice flour
1 teaspoon baking soda
½ cup carob chips (unsweetened)
dash allspice (optional)

Oil two baking sheets and preheat oven to 375 degrees F. In a medium-size mixing bowl, combine the oil, maple syrup, and vanilla. Beat the egg and stir into the oil mixture. Gradually stir in flour and baking soda to form a stiff batter. Fold in carob chips and drop the batter onto the baking sheets by the teaspoon. Bake for 10 to 15 minutes, until cookies are lightly browned. Remove from oven and cool.

Makes 3½ to 4 dozen.

KIFTA

2 pounds finely ground lamb meat
1 large onion, finely chopped
2 to 2½ teaspoons salt
1½ teaspoons pepper and allspice
1 cup parsley, finely chopped
½ cup lemon juice

Mix all of the ingredients thoroughly (using a meat grinder, if you have one). Reserve parsley and lemon juice.

To barbecue: Take portions of meat and mold on skewers, making sure it is held firmly.

To broil: Take portions of meat and mold into rolls, lengthwise, 3 inches long. Place on a broiling pan and broil in a preheated oven at 500 degrees F. When brown on one side, broil for a few minutes on the other side.

Serve hot. Sprinkle with lemon juice and garnish with parsley.

Type O
Supplement Advisory

THE ROLE OF SUPPLEMENTS—be they vitamins, minerals, or herbs—is to add the nutrients that are lacking in your diet and to provide extra protection where you need it. The supplement focus for Type Os is:

- Supercharging the metabolism
- Increasing blood-clotting activity
- Preventing inflammation
- Stabilizing the thyroid

The following recommendations emphasize the supplements that help meet these goals, and also warn against the supplements that can be counterproductive or dangerous for Type Os.

Certain common vitamins and minerals are so abundant in Type O foods that they are normally not needed in supplement form. These include vitamin C and iron—although it won't hurt you to take a 500 mg vitamin C supplement every day. Vitamin D supplements are not needed. Many foods are vitamin D fortified, and your best source of all is the natural light of the sun.

All of these recommendations are based on your adherence to the Type O Diet.

Beneficial

VITAMIN B

My father found that Type Os did well on a high-potency vitamin B complex. There's good reason. Type Os tend to have sluggish metabolisms—a holdover from your ancestors' efforts to conserve energy during periods when food was not readily available. Since modern Type Os experience very different conditions, they don't need this conserving effect, but it remains in your blood type memory. A vitamin B complex can have the effect of supercharging your metabolic processes.

Type Os on the correct diet almost never require special vitamin B-12 or folic acid supplementation. I have, however, successfully treated depression, hyperactivity, and attention deficit disorder (ADD) in many Type Os by using high doses of folic acid and vitamin B-12 in conjunction with the Type O Diet and exercise program. Those vitamins are responsible for the development of DNA.

If you wish to experiment with a high-potency vitamin B complex, make sure it is free of fillers and binders. Improper binding and compressing can make the pill difficult to absorb in your system. Also avoid using a formula that contains yeast or wheat germ.

Finally, eat plenty of vitamin B–rich foods.

Best B-Rich Foods for Type Os:

meat	nuts
liver, kidney,	recommended
muscle meats	dark green,
*eggs	leafy vegetables
fish	fruit

in moderation

VITAMIN K

Type Os have lower levels of several blood-clotting factors, which lead to bleeding disorders. Be sure you have plenty of vitamin K in your diet. Since it is generally not recommended as a supplement, pay attention to the foods you eat and choose those that are high in this essential Type O nutrient.

Best K-Rich Foods for Type Os:

> liver
> egg yolks
> green leafy vegetables—kale, spinach, and Swiss chard

CALCIUM

Type Os should continually supplement their diet with calcium, since the Type O Diet does not include dairy products which are the best source of this mineral. With the Type O tendency to develop inflammatory joint problems and arthritis, the need for consistent calcium supplementation becomes clear.

Calcium supplementation in high doses (600–1,100 mg elemental calcium) is probably desirable for all Type Os, but it is especially beneficial for Type O children during their growth periods (two to five and nine to sixteen), and for post-menopausal women.

Although the non-dairy sources of calcium are not as beneficial, Type Os should employ them as mainstays of their diets.

Best Calcium-Rich Foods for Type Os

> sardines (unboned)
> canned salmon (unboned)
> broccoli
> collard greens

IODINE

Type Os tend to have unstable thyroid metabolisms, due to a lack of iodine. This causes many side effects, including weight gain, fluid retention, and fatigue. Iodine is the key element necessary for the production of thyroid hormone. Although iodine supplements are not recommended, adequate amounts of iodine can be found in the Type O Diet.

Best Iodine-Rich Foods for Type Os

seafood (especially saltwater fish)
kelp (seaweed)
*iodized salt

*in moderation

MANGANESE [*with caution*]
It is difficult for Type Os to get manganese in their diet because manganese is found primarily in whole grains and legumes. For the most part this isn't a problem, and manganese supplementation is rarely recommended. However, a surprising amount of chronic joint pain (especially in the lower back and knees) in Type O patients has been helped with a short period of manganese supplementation. Never do this on your own! Manganese toxicity can result from inappropriate administration, and it should be used only under a physician's supervision.

Herbs/Phytochemicals: Recommended for Type Os

LICORICE *(Glycyrrhiza glabra)*. The high stomach acid typical of Type Os can lead to stomach irritations and ulcers. A licorice preparation called DGL (de-glycyrrhizinated licorice) can reduce your discomfort and aid healing. DGL is widely available in health food stores as a pleasant-tasting powder or in the form of lozenges. Unlike most ulcer medicines, DGL actually heals the stomach lining, in addition to protecting it from stomach acids. Avoid crude licorice preparations, as they contain a component of the plant that can cause elevated blood pressure. This component has been removed in DGL.

BLADDER WRACK *(Fucus vesiculosus).* Bladder wrack (from kelp) is an excellent nutrient for Type Os. This herb, actually a seaweed, has some interesting components, including iodine and large amounts of the sugar fucose. As you may recall, fucose is the basic building sugar of the O antigen. The fucose found in bladder wrack helps protect the intestinal lining of Type Os—especially from the ulcer-causing bacteria, *H. pylori,* which attaches itself to the fucose lining the stomach of Type Os. The fucose in bladder wrack acts on H. pylori much as dust would on a piece of adhesive tape: clogging the suction cups on the bacteria, preventing it from attaching to the stomach.

I have also found that bladder wrack is very effective as an aid to weight control for Type Os—especially those who suffer thyroid dysfunctions. The fucose in bladder wrack seems to help normalize the sluggish metabolic rate and produce weight loss. (Note, however, that although bladder wrack has a time-honored reputation as an aid to weight loss for Type Os, it does not work that way for the other blood types.)

PANCREATIC ENZYMES. If you are a Type O who is not used to a high-protein diet, I suggest you take a pancreatic enzyme with large meals for a while, or at least until your system begins to adjust to the more concentrated proteins. Pancreatic enzyme supplements are available at many health food stores, usually in the 4x strength.

Avoid

VITAMIN A
Since your blood type is prone to slower clotting, I would not recommend that Type Os take vitamin A supplements derived from fish oils without first checking with a doctor. These supplements can enhance blood thinning. Instead, take advantage of the rich sources of vitamin A or beta-carotene in your diet.

A-Rich Foods Acceptable for Type Os

>yellow, orange, and recommended dark, leafy green
>vegetables

VITAMIN E

Likewise, I would not recommend vitamin E supplements for Type Os because they might also complicate Type O tendencies toward slower blood clotting. Instead, derive vitamin E from foods in your diet.

E-Rich Foods Acceptable for Type Os

>vegetable oils
>liver
>nuts
>recommended leafy green vegetables

Type O
Stress/Exercise Profile

THE ABILITY to reverse the negative effects of stress lives in your blood type. As we discussed in chapter 3, stress is not in itself the problem; it's how you respond to stress. Each blood type has a distinct, genetically programmed instinct for overcoming stress.

If you are Type O, you have the immediate and physical response of our hunter ancestors: stress goes directly to your muscles. Your blood type carries a patterned alarm response that permits explosions of intense physical energy.

When you encounter stress, your body takes over. As your adrenal glands pump their chemicals into your bloodstream, you become tremendously charged up. Given a physical release at this time, any bad stress you are experiencing may be converted into a positive experience.

Healthy Type Os are meant to release the built-up hormonal forces through vigorous and intense physical exercise. Their systems are literally suited for it.

Exercise is especially critical to the health of Type Os, because the impact of stress is direct and physical.

Not only does a regular intense exercise program elevate your spirits, it enables the Type O to maintain weight control, emotional balance, and a strong self-image. Type Os respond well to heavy exercise—in nearly every way.

Type Os who want to lose weight must participate in highly physical exercise. That is because this type of exercise makes the muscle tissue more acidic and produces a higher rate of fat-burning activity. Acidic muscle tissue is the result of ketosis, which, as we have discussed, was the key to the success of our Type O ancestors. I'd dare to say that there wasn't one overweight Cro-Magnon on the planet!

Type Os who do not express their physical natures with appropriate activity in response to stress are eventually overwhelmed during the exhaustion stage of the stress response. This exhaustion stage is characterized by a variety of psychological manifestations caused by a slower rate of metabolism, such as depression, fatigue, or insomnia. If there is no change, you will leave yourself vulnerable to a number of inflammatory and autoimmune disorders, such as arthritis and asthma, as well as to consistent weight gain and eventual obesity.

The following exercises are recommended for Type Os. Pay special attention to the length of the sessions. To achieve a consistent metabolic effect, you have to get your heart rate up.

You can mix any of these exercises, but be sure you do one or several of them at least four times a week for the best results.

EXERCISE	DURATION	FREQUENCY
AEROBICS	40–60 min.	3–4x week
SWIMMING	30–45 min..	3–4x week
JOGGING	30 min.	3–4x week
WEIGHT TRAINING	30 min.	3x week
TREADMILL	30 min.	3x week

STAIR CLIMBING	20–30 min.	3–4x week
MARTIAL ARTS	60 min.	2–3x week
CONTACT SPORTS	60 min.	2–3x week
CALISTHENICS	30–45 min.	3x week
CYCLING	30 min.	3x week
BRISK WALKING	30–40 min.	5x week
DANCING	40–60 min.	3x week
IN-LINE OR ROLLER SKATING	30 min.	3–4x week

Type O
Exercise Guidelines

THE THREE COMPONENTS of a high-intensity exercise program are the warm-up period, the aerobic exercise period, and the cooldown period. A warm-up is very important to prevent injuries, because it brings blood to the muscles, readying them for exercise, whether it is walking, running, biking, swimming, or playing a sport. A warm-up should include stretching and flexibility moves, to prevent tears in the muscles and tendons.

The exercise can be divided into two basic types: isometric exercises, in which stress is created in stationary muscles; and isotonic exercises, such as calisthenics, running, or swimming, which produce muscle tension through a range of movement. Isometric exercises can be used to tone up specific muscles, which can be further strengthened by active isotonic exercise. Isometrics may be performed by pushing or pulling an immovable object or by contracting or tightening opposing muscles.

To achieve maximum cardiovascular benefits from aerobic exercise, you must elevate your heartbeat to approximately 70 percent of your maximum heart rate. Once that elevated rate is achieved during exercise, continue exercising to maintain that rate for thirty minutes. This regimen should be repeated at least three times each week.

To calculate your maximum heart rate:

1. Subtract your age from 220.
2. Multiply the difference by 70 percent (.70). If you are over sixty years of age, or in poor physical condition, multiply the remainder by 60 percent (.60).
3. Multiply the remainder by 50 percent (.50). For example, a healthy fifty-year-old woman would subtract 50 from 220, for a maximum heart rate of 170. Multiplying 170 by .70 would give her 119 beats per minute, which is the top level she should strive for. Multiplying 170 by .50 would give her 85 beats per minute, the lowest number in her range.

Active, healthy individuals under forty and persons under sixty with a low cardiovascular risk can choose their own exercise program from among the recommendations listed.

Remember, your goal is to counter stress with action. Remarkably, for Type Os, the best antidote to fatigue and depression is physical work. Think of your metabolism as a fire. You start a fire first by using little pieces of wood called kindling, and then gradually adding larger and larger pieces of wood until you have an inferno. If you are too tired to imagine doing aerobics for forty-five minutes or an hour, start doing something! As you feel better, add more. At the end, your stress levels will be reduced, your mood will be better, and you'll have renewed energy.

A Final Note:
The Personality Question

EVERY PERSON with Type O blood carries a genetic memory of strength, endurance, self-reliance, daring, intuition, and an innate optimism. The original Type Os were the epitome of focus, drive, and a strong sense of self-preservation. They believed in themselves. It's a good thing, too, or we might not be here.

If you are a Type O, you may be able to appreciate this inheritance because the things that make you healthy, inspire you, and energize you are very similar to what influenced your ancestors. You're hardy and strong, fueled by a high-protein diet. You respond best to heavy physical exercise—in fact, you become depressed, despondent, and overweight when you are deprived of it.

Perhaps you have also inherited the drive to succeed and the leadership qualities of Type Os—strong, certain and powerful—blushing with good health and optimism.

Former president Ronald Reagan is a Type O who fits the mold quite well. His administration was characterized by a surety, evenness, and an unflagging optimism about the future. You never felt that Reagan suffered much in the way of self-doubt. He forged ahead, for good or ill. He was also a risk taker, as is the way of Type Os. People used to call him the "Teflon president" because he was never felled by the risks he took.

Of course, Reagan didn't exhibit (at least publicly) the sharp, uncompromising, almost brutish style of some leaders. For example, it's not terribly surprising that some famous mafiosos have been Type Os. Al Capone was a Type O. Now, there's an example of leadership taken to the extreme.

And speaking of risk takers, the penultimate gambler, Jimmy the Greek, was Type O. So is former Soviet president Mikhail Gorbachev—one of the greatest risk takers of modern times.

Great Britain's Queen Elizabeth II is a Type O, as is her son Charles, the Prince of Wales. I find it interesting that the House of Windsor has a history of people with bleeding disorders. Perhaps there's a Type O connection.

FIVE

Blood Type

A

*P*lan

TYPE A: *The Cultivator*

- THE FIRST VEGETARIAN
- REAPS WHAT HE SOWS
- SENSITIVE DIGESTIVE TRACT
- TOLERANT IMMUNE SYSTEM
- ADAPTS WELL TO SETTLED DIETARY AND ENVIRONMENTAL CONDITIONS
- RESPONDS BEST TO STRESS WITH CALMING ACTION
- REQUIRES AGRARIAN DIET TO STAY LEAN AND PRODUCTIVE

The Type A Diet

TYPE As flourish on vegetarian diets—the inheritance of their more settled and less warlike farmer ancestors. If you are an average American with Type A blood, you might find it too big an adjustment to move away from the typical meat-and-potato fare to soy proteins, grains, and vegetables. Likewise, you may find it difficult to eliminate overly processed and refined foods, since our civilized diets are increasingly composed of convenient toxins in brightly wrapped packages. But it is particularly important for sensitive Type As to get their foods in as natural a state as possible: fresh, pure, and organic.

I can't emphasize enough how critical this dietary adjustment can be to the sensitive immune system of Type A. As you will see in chapter 9, Type As are biologically predisposed to heart disease, cancer, and diabetes. In other words, these are your risk factors. But they need not be your destiny. If you follow this diet, you can supercharge your immune system and potentially short-circuit the development of life-threatening diseases. A positive aspect of your genetic ancestry is your ability to utilize the best nature has to offer. It will be your challenge to relearn what your blood already knows.

The Weight-Loss Factor

YOU WILL NATURALLY be thinner on the Type A Diet. If you are accustomed to eating meat, you'll lose weight rather rapidly in the beginning as you eliminate the toxic foods from your diet.

In many ways, Type A is the exact opposite of Type O when it comes to metabolism. While animal foods speed up the Type O metabolic rate and make it more efficient, they have a very different effect on Type As. Perhaps you have already noted that when you eat red meat, you feel sluggish and less energized than when you eat vegetable proteins. Some Type As experience

fluid retention as their digestive systems slowly process the un-
wieldy foods. Type Os burn their meat as fuel; Type As ultimately
store meat as fat. The reason for the difference is stomach acid.
While Type Os have high stomach-acid content, which promotes
easy digestion of meat, Type As have low stomach-acid content—
an adaptation of their ancestors who survived on an agrarian diet.

Dairy foods are also poorly digested by Type As, and they pro-
voke insulin reactions—another factor in metabolic slowdowns.
In addition, dairy foods are very high in saturated fats, the kind
that compromise the heart and lead to obesity and diabetes.

Wheat is a mixed factor in the Type A Diet. While Type As
may eat wheat, they have to be careful not to eat too much of it or
their muscle tissue will become overly acidic. Unlike Type Os,
who thrive on slightly acidic tissue, Type As can't utilize the energy as quickly, and calorie metabolism is inhibited. This particular food reaction is a good example of how different foods react
in different ways depending on your blood type. Wheat is alkaline in Type Os and acidic in Type As.

In addition to eating a wide variety of healthy, low-fat foods
and balancing vegetables and grains, Type As need to highlight
certain foods for their beneficial or hindering effects. Here's a
quick guide:

FOODS THAT ENCOURAGE WEIGHT GAIN

MEAT	*poorly digested*
	stored as fat
	increases digestive toxins
DAIRY FOODS	*inhibit nutrient metabolism*
	increases mucous secretions
KIDNEY BEANS	*interfere with digestive enzymes*
	slow metabolic rate
LIMA BEANS	*interfere with digestive enzymes*
	slow metabolic rate
WHEAT (IN	*inhibits insulin effciency*
OVERABUNDANCE)	*impairs calorie utilization*

FOODS THAT ENCOURAGE WEIGHT LOSS

VEGETABLE OILS   *aid efficient digestion*
prevent fluid retention
SOY FOODS   *aid efficient digestion*
metabolize quickly
optimize immune function
VEGETABLES   *aid efficient metabolism*
increase intestinal mobility
PINEAPPLE   *increases calorie utilization*
increases intestinal mobility

INCORPORATE THESE GUIDELINES INTO THE TOTAL PICTURE OF THE
TYPE A DIET, WHICH FOLLOWS.

Meats and Poultry

BLOOD TYPE A		WEEKLY ▪ IF YOUR ANCESTRY IS		
Food	*Portion*	*African*	*Caucasian*	*Asian*
LEAN RED MEATS	4–6 OZ. *(men)* 2–5 OZ. *(women and children)*	0–1X	0X	0–1X
POULTRY	4–6 OZ. *(men)* 2–5 OZ. *(women and children)*	0–3X	0–3X	1–4X

*The portion recommendations are merely guidelines that can help refine your diet according to ancestral propensities.

To receive the greatest benefits, Type As should eliminate all meats from their diet. Let's be realistic, however. The Western diet is still resolutely protein-driven. The trend in fast-food restaurants seems to be bigger, with more fat and calories than ever before. But, no matter the current trend, I urge you to look at the Type A Diet guidelines with an open mind. This is a way you can begin reducing Type A risk factors for heart disease and cancer in your diet.

Having said that, let me acknowledge that it will probably take time for you to convert to a totally vegetarian diet. Begin by substituting fish for meat several times a week. When you do eat meat, choose the leanest cuts you can find; poultry is preferable to red meat. Prepare meat by broiling or baking.

Stay completely away from processed meat products such as ham, frankfurters, and cold cuts. They contain nitrites, which promote stomach cancer in people with low levels of stomach acid—a Type A trait.

Neutral

Chicken
Cornish hens
Turkey

Avoid

Bacon	Ham	Pheasant
Beef	Heart	Pork
Beef ground	Lamb	Rabbit
Buffalo	Liver	Veal
Duck	Mutton	Venison
Goose	Partridge	Quail

Seafood

BLOOD TYPE A		WEEKLY ▪ IF YOUR ANCESTRY IS		
Food	*Portion*	*African*	*Caucasian*	*Asian*
ALL RECOMMENDED SEAFOOD	4–6 OZ.	0–3X	1–4X	1–4X

Type As can eat seafood in modest quantities three or four times a week, but should avoid white fish such as sole and flounder. They contain a lectin that can irritate the Type A digestive tract.

If you are a Type A woman with a family history of breast cancer, consider introducing snails into your diet. The edible snail *Helix pomatia* contains a powerful lectin that specifically agglutinates and is drawn to mutated Type A cells for two of the most common forms of breast cancer, as you will see in chapter 10. This is a positive kind of agglutination; this lectin gets rid of sick cells.

Seafood should be baked, broiled, or poached to achieve its full nutritional value.

Highly Beneficial

CARP	RED SNAPPER	SILVER PERCH
COD	RAINBOW	SNAIL
GROUPER	TROUT	WHITEFISH
MACKEREL	SALMON	YELLOW
MONKFISH	SARDINE	PERCH
PICKEREL	SEA TROUT	

Neutral

Abalone	Sailfish	Swordfish
Albacore (Tuna)	Sea bass	Weakfish
Mahimahi	Shark	White perch
Ocean perch	Smelt	Yellowtail
Pike	Snapper	
Porgy	Sturgeon	

Avoid

Anchovy	Bluefish	Caviar
Barracuda	Bluegill bass	Clam
Beluga	Catfish	Conch

Crab	Herring (fresh)	Shad
Crayfish	Herring (pickled)	Shrimp
Eel	Lobster	Sole
Flounder	Lox (smoked	Squid (calamari)
Frog	salmon)	Striped bass
Gray sole	Mussels	Tilefish
Haddock	Octopus	Turtle
Hake	Oysters	
Halibut	Scallop	

Eggs and Dairy

BLOOD TYPE A		WEEKLY ▪ IF YOUR ANCESTRY IS		
Food	*Portion*	*African*	*Caucasian*	*Asian*
EGGS	1 EGG	1–3X	1–3X	1–3X
CHEESES	2 OZ.	1–3X	2–4X	0
YOGURT	4–6 OZ.	0	1–3X	0–3X
MILK	4–6 OZ.	0	0–4X	0

Type As can tolerate small amounts of fermented dairy products, but should avoid anything made with whole milk, and also limit egg consumption to occasional organically grown eggs. This will take some planning, as the Western diet is egg, butter, and cream oriented—cakes, pies, cookies, and ice cream being the big favorites.

Your Type A choices should be yogurt, kefir, nonfat sour cream, and cultured dairy products. Raw goat's milk is a good substitute for whole milk. And, of course, soy milk and soy cheeses are excellent substitutes, and are very good for Type As.

Most dairy products are not digestible for Type As—for the simple reason that Type A blood creates antibodies to the primary sugar in whole milk—D-galactosamine. As you'll remember from chapter 2, D-galactosamine is the essential sugar that, along with fucose, forms the Type B antigen. Since the Type A immune system is designed to reject anything B-like, the antibodies it creates to ward off B antigens will also reject whole-milk products.

If you are a Type A allergy sufferer or are experiencing respiratory problems, be aware that dairy products greatly increase the amount of mucus you secrete. Type As normally produce more mucus than the other blood types, probably because they need the extra protection it provides their somewhat too friendly immune systems. However, too much mucus can be harmful, since various bacteria tend to live off it. An overabundance of mucus inevitably leads to allergic responses, infections, and respiratory problems. This is another good reason to limit your intake of dairy foods.

Highly Beneficial

SOYA CHEESE*
SOY MILK*

Good dairy alternatives

Neutral

Farmer	Kefir	String cheese
Feta	Mozzarella,	Yogurt
Goat cheese	low fat	Yogurt with fruit
Goat milk	Ricotta, low fat	Yogurt, frozen

Avoid

American cheese	Camembert	Cream cheese
Blue cheese	Casein	Edam
Brie	Cheddar	Emmenthal
Butter	Colby	Gouda
Buttermilk	Cottage	Gruyère

Ice cream	Parmesan	Skim or 2% milk
Jarlsberg	Provolone	Swiss
Monterey jack	Neufchatel	Whey
Munster	Sherbet	Whole milk

Oils and Fats

BLOOD TYPE A		WEEKLY ▪ IF YOUR ANCESTRY IS		
Food	*Portion*	*African*	*Caucasian*	*Asian*
OILS	1 TABLESPOON	3–8X	2–6X	2–6X

Type As need very little fat to function well, but a tablespoon of olive oil on salads or steamed vegetables every day will aid in digestion and elimination. As a monounsaturated fat, olive oil also has a positive effect on your heart and may actually reduce cholesterol.

The lectins in oils like corn and safflower oil cause problems in the Type A digestive tract—quite the opposite effect of the beneficial oils.

Of course, there are only two oils that are highly beneficial, and frankly, olive oil is far tastier and better suited for cooking than linseed oil.

Highly Beneficial

LINSEED (FLAXSEED) OIL
OLIVE OIL

Neutral

Canola oil
Cod liver oil

Avoid

Corn oil   Safflower oil
Cottonseed oil   Sesame oil
Peanut oil

Nuts and Seeds

BLOOD TYPE A		WEEKLY ■ IF YOUR ANCESTRY IS		
Food	*Portion*	*African*	*Caucasian*	*Asian*
NUTS AND SEEDS	SMALL HANDFUL	4–6X	2–5X	4–6X
NUT BUTTERS	TABLESPOON	3–5X	1–4X	2–4X

Many nuts and seeds, such as pumpkin and sunflower seeds, almonds, and walnuts can provide positive supplementation for the Type A Diet. Since Type As eat very little animal protein, nuts and seeds supply an important protein component. Peanuts are the most beneficial. Eat them often because they contain a cancer-fighting lectin. Also eat the peanut skins (not the shells). Pumpkin seeds are also highly beneficial.

If you are Type A and have gallbladder problems, limit yourself to small amounts of nut butters instead of whole nuts.

Highly Beneficial

PEANUTS
PEANUT BUTTER
PUMPKIN SEEDS

Neutral

Almond butter   Nuts, filberts   Nuts, macadamia
Nuts, almonds   Nuts, hickory   Nuts, pignola (pine)
Nuts, chestnuts   Nuts, litchi   Poppy seeds

Sesame seeds   Sunflower butter
Sesame butter   Sunflower seeds
  (tahini)   Walnuts

<u>Avoid</u>

Brazil nuts
Cashews
Pistachios

Beans and Legumes

BLOOD TYPE A		WEEKLY ▪ IF YOUR ANCESTRY IS		
Food	*Portion*	*African*	*Caucasian*	*Asian*
ALL RECOMMENDED BEANS AND LEGUMES	I CUP, DRY	4–7X	3–6X	2–5X

Type As thrive on the vegetable proteins found in beans and legumes. Along with your friend the soybean, and all of its related products, many beans and legumes provide a nutritious source of protein. Be aware, however, that not all beans and legumes are good for you. Some, like the kidney, lima, navy, and garbanzo, contain a lectin that can cause a decrease in insulin production, which is often a factor in both obesity and diabetes.

Highly Beneficial

BEANS, ADUKE   BEANS, PINTO   LENTILS, GREEN
BEANS, AZUKI   BEANS, RED SOY   LENTILS, RED
BEANS, BLACK   LENTILS,   PEAS, BLACK-
BEANS, GREEN   DOMESTIC   EYED

Neutral

Beans, broad	Beans, snap	Peas, pods
Beans, cannellini	Beans, string	Peas, snow
Beans, fava	Beans, white	
Beans, jicama	Peas, green	

Avoid

Beans, copper	Beans, navy
Beans, garbanzo	Beans, red
Beans, kidney	Beans, tamarind
Beans, lima	

Cereals

BLOOD TYPE A		WEEKLY ∎ IF YOUR ANCESTRY IS		
Food	*Portion*	*African*	*Caucasian*	*Asian*
WHOLE GRAINS	I CUP, DRY	6–10X	5–9X	4–8X
PASTAS	I CUP, DRY	3–5X	4–6X	3–5X

Type As generally do well on cereals and grains, and you can eat these foods one or more times a day. Select the more concentrated whole grains instead of instant and processed cereals. Introduce millet, soy wheat, cornmeal, and whole oats into your diet.

Type As with a pronounced mucus condition caused by asthma or frequent infections should limit wheat consumption, as wheat causes mucus production. You'll have to experiment for yourself to determine how much wheat you can eat.

Wheat-eating Type As must be sure to balance their intake of acid-forming wheat with alkaline foods (see fruits). We're not talking about stomach acid here, but the acid/alkaline balance in your muscle tissues. Type As do best when their tissues are slightly alkaline—in direct contrast with Type Os. While the inner kernel of wheat grain is alkaline in Type Os, it becomes acidic in Type As.

Highly Beneficial

AMARANTH
BUCKWHEAT

Neutral

Barley	Kamut	Rice, puffed
Cornflakes	Millet, puffed	Rice bran
Cornmeal	Oat bran	Spelt
Cream of rice	Oatmeal	

Avoid

Cream of wheat	Granola	Seven grain
Familia	Grape nuts	Shredded wheat
Farina	Wheat germ	Wheat bran

Breads and Muffins

BLOOD TYPE A	DAILY ■ IF YOUR ANCESTRY IS			
Food	Portion	African	Caucasian	Asian
BREADS, CRACKERS	I SLICE	2–4X	3–5X	2–4X
MUFFINS	I MUFFIN	IX	1–2X	IX

The Type A guidelines for breads and muffins are similar to those for cereals and grains. They are generally favorable foods, but if you produce excessive mucus or are overweight, these conditions make whole wheat inadvisable. Soy and rice flour are good substitutes for you. However, be aware that sprouted wheat breads sold commercially often contain small amounts of sprouted wheat and are basically whole wheat breads. Read the ingredient labels. Although Essene and Ezekiel breads (found in health food stores) are sprouted wheat breads, the gluten lectin is destroyed in the sprouting process.

Highly Beneficial

ESSENE BREAD	RICE CAKES	SPROUTED
EZEKIEL	SOYA FLOUR	WHEAT BREAD
BREAD	BREAD	

Neutral

Brown rice bread	Ideal Flat Bread	Rye Crisps
Corn muffins	Millet	Rye Vita
Fin Crisp	Oat bran muffins	Spelt bread
Gluten-free bread	Rye bread, 100%	Wasa bread

Avoid

Durum wheat	Matzos, wheat	Wheat bran
English muffins	Multi-grain	muffins
High-protein	bread	Whole wheat
bread	Pumpernickel	bread

Grains and Pasta

BLOOD TYPE A		WEEKLY ■ IF YOUR ANCESTRY IS		
Food	Portion	African	Caucasian	Asian
GRAINS	1 CUP, DRY	2–3X	2–4X	2–4X
PASTAS	1 CUP, DRY	2–3X	2–4X	2–4X

Type As have a wonderful cornucopia of choices in grains and pastas. These foods are excellent sources of vegetable protein. They can provide many of the nutrients that the Type A is no longer receiving from animal proteins. Stay away from processed products, such as frozen meals, prepared noodles with sauces, or packaged rice-and-vegetable combinations; instead, gain the full nutritional benefits from whole-grain products. Bake your own cakes, prepare your own pasta, or steam your own rice, using the purest ingredients.

Highly Beneficial

BUCKWHEAT	NOODLES, SOBA
FLOUR, OAT	PASTA,
FLOUR, RICE	ARTICHOKE
FLOUR, RYE	

Neutral

Couscous	Flour, gluten	Quinoa
Flour, barley	Flour, graham	Rice, basmati
Flour, bulgur wheat	Flour, spelt	Rice, brown
Flour, durum wheat	Flour, sprouted wheat	Rice, white
	Noodles, spelt	Rice, wild

Avoid

Flour, white	Pasta, semolina
Flour, whole wheat	Pasta, spinach

Vegetables

BLOOD TYPE A		DAILY ■ IF YOUR ANCESTRY IS		
Food	*Portion*	*African*	*Caucasian*	*Asian*
VEGETABLES, RAW	1 CUP, COOKED	3–6X	2–5X	2–5X
VEGETABLES, COOKED	1 CUP, COOKED	1–4X	3–6X	3–6X
SOY PRODUCTS	6–8 OUNCES	4–6X WEEK	4–6X WEEK	5–7X WEEK

Vegetables are vital to the Type A Diet, providing minerals, enzymes, and antioxidants. Eat your vegetables in as natural a state as possible (raw or steamed) to preserve their full benefits.

Most vegetables are available to Type As, but there are a few caveats: peppers aggravate the delicate Type A stomach, as do the molds in fermented olives. Type As are also very sensitive to the lectins in domestic potatoes, sweet potatoes, yams, and cabbage. Avoid tomatoes, as their lectins have a strongly deleterious effect on the Type A digestive tract. Tomatoes are a rare food— what is called a panhemaglutinan. That means its lectins agglutinate in every blood type. However, Type O doesn't produce antibodies to tomatoes, and can eat them, as can Type AB. They're very bad for Type As and Type Bs, though.

Broccoli is highly recommended for its antioxidant benefits. Antioxidants strengthen the immune system and prevent abnormal cell division. Other vegetables that are excellent for Type As are carrots, collard greens, kale, pumpkin, and spinach.

Use plenty of garlic. It's a natural antibiotic and immune-system booster, and it's good for your blood. Every blood type benefits from the use of garlic, but perhaps Type As benefit most of all, because their immune systems are vulnerable to a number of diseases that garlic ameliorates. Yellow onions are very good immune boosters, too. They contain an antioxidant called quercetin.

And, of course, tofu is the staple of the Type A Diet. Tofu is a nutritionally complete food that is both filling and inexpensive. Many people in Western societies have an automatic aversion to tofu. I think the real problem with tofu is the way it is usually displayed in the markets, in big plastic tubs of cold water. It doesn't look very appetizing. I've found that tofu displayed this way isn't as good as tofu that is refrigerated. Also, try to purchase tofu in health food stores, where it is likely to be fresher than in supermarkets. Tofu is tasteless; it takes on the flavors of vegetables and spices used in cooking. The best way to prepare it is in a stir-fry with vegetables and flavoring such as garlic, ginger, and soy sauce.

Highly Beneficial

ARTICHOKE, DOMESTIC	ESCAROLE	ONIONS, YELLOW
	GARLIC	PARSLEY
ARTICHOKE, JERUSALEM	HORSERADISH	PARSNIPS
	KALE	PUMPKIN
BEET LEAVES	KOHLRABI	SPINACH
BROCCOLI	LEEK	SPROUTS,
CARROTS	LETTUCE,	ALFALFA
CHICORY	ROMAINE	SWISS CHARD
COLLARD GREENS	OKRA	TEMPEH
	ONIONS, RED	TOFU
DANDELION	ONIONS, SPANISH	TURNIPS

Neutral

Arugula	Cauliflower	Daikon radish
Asparagus	Celery	Endive
Avocado	Chervil	Fennel
Bamboo shoots	Coriander	Fiddlehead ferns
Beets	Corn, white	Lettuce, Bibb
Bok choy	Corn, yellow	Lettuce, Boston
Caraway	Cucumber	Lettuce, iceberg

Lettuce, mesclun

Mushroom, abalone

Mushroom, enoki

Mushroom, maitake

Mushroom, Portobello

Mushroom, shiitake

Mushroom, tree oyster

Mustard greens

Olives, green

Onions, green

Radicchio

Radishes

Rappini

Rutabaga

Scallion

Seaweed

Shallots

Sprouts, Brussels

Sprouts, mung

Sprouts, radish

Squash, all types

Water chestnut

Watercress

Zucchini

Avoid

Cabbage, Chinese

Cabbage, red

Cabbage, white

Eggplant

Lima beans

Mushroom, domestic

Olives, black

Olives, Greek

Olives, Spanish

Peppers, green

Peppers, jalapeno

Peppers, red

Peppers, yellow

Potatoes, sweet

Potatoes, red

Potatoes, white

Tomatoes

Yams

Fruits

BLOOD TYPE A	DAILY ■ ALL ANCESTRAL TYPES
Food	*Portion*
ALL RECOMMENDED FRUITS	1 FRUIT OR 3–5 OZ. 3–4X

Type As should eat fruits three times a day. Most fruits are allowable, although you should try to emphasize the more alkaline ones, such as berries and plums, which can help to balance the grains that are acid forming in your muscle tissues. Melons are also alkaline, but their high mold counts make them hard for Type As to digest. Cantaloupe and honeydew melons should be avoided altogether, since they have the highest mold counts. Other melons (listed as neutral) can be eaten occasionally.

Type As don't do well on tropical fruits such as mangoes and papaya. Although these fruits contain a digestive enzyme that is good for the other blood types, it doesn't work in the Type A digestive tract. Pineapple, on the other hand, is an excellent digestive aid for Type As.

Oranges also should be avoided, even though they may well be among your favorites. Oranges are a stomach irritant for Type As, and they also interfere with the absorption of important minerals. Lest you get confused, let me clarify that the acid/alkaline reaction happens two different ways—in the stomach and in the muscle tissues. When I say that acidic oranges are a stomach irritant for Type As, I'm talking about the stomach irritation they can cause in the sensitive, alkaline Type A stomach. Although stomach acid is generally low in Type As and could use a boost, oranges irritate the delicate stomach lining. Grapefruit is closely related to oranges and is also an acidic fruit, but it has positive effects on the Type A stomach, exhibiting alkaline tendencies after digestion. Lemons are also excellent for Type As, helping to aid digestion and clear mucus from the system.

Since vitamin C is an important antioxidant, especially for stomach cancer prevention, eat other vitamin C–rich fruits, such as grapefruit or kiwi.

The banana lectin interferes with Type A digestion. I recommend substituting other high-potassium fruits such as apricots, figs, and certain melons.

Highly Beneficial

APRICOTS	CRANBERRIES	PINEAPPLE
BLACKBERRIES	FIGS, DRIED	PLUMS, DARK
BLUEBERRIES	FIGS, FRESH	PLUMS, GREEN
BOYSENBERRIES	GRAPEFRUIT	PLUMS, RED
CHERRIES	LEMONS	PRUNES

Neutral

Apples	Kumquat	Peaches
Currants, black	Limes	Pears
Currants, red	Loganberries	Persimmons
Dates	Melon, canang	Pomegranates
Elderberries	Melon, casaba	Prickly pears
Gooseberries	Melon, Christmas	Raisins
Grapes, black	Melon, Crenshaw	Raspberries
Grapes, Concord	Melon, musk	Star fruit,
Grapes, green	Melon, Spanish	carambola
Grapes, red	Melon,	Strawberries
Guava	watermelon	
Kiwi	Nectarines	

Avoid

Bananas	Melon, honeydew	Rhubarb
Coconuts	Oranges	Tangerines
Mangoes	Papayas	
Melon,	Plantains	
cantaloupe		

Juices and Fluids

BLOOD TYPE A		DAILY ▪ ALL ANCESTRAL TYPES
Food	*Portion*	
ALL RECOMMENDED JUICES	8 OZ.	4–5X
LEMON AND WATER	8 OZ.	1X (IN MORNING)
WATER	8 OZ.	1–3X

Type As should start every day with a small glass of warm water into which they have squeezed the juice of one-half lemon. This will help you reduce the mucus that has accumulated overnight in the more sluggish Type A digestive tract and stimulate normal elimination.

Alkaline fruit juices, such as black cherry juice concentrate diluted with water, should be consumed in preference to high-sugar juices, which are more acid forming.

Highly Beneficial

APRICOT	GRAPEFRUIT
CARROT	PINEAPPLE
CELERY	PRUNE
CHERRY, BLACK	WATER (WITH LEMON)

Neutral

Apple	Grape
Apple cider	Vegetable juice
Cabbage	(corresponding
Cucumber	to highlighted
Cranberry	vegetables)

Avoid

Orange
Papaya
Tomato

Spices

Type As should view spices as more than just flavor enhancers. The right combination of spices can be powerful immune-system boosters. For example, soy-based spices such as tamari, miso, and soy sauce are tremendously beneficial for Type As. If you're concerned about sodium intake, all of these products are available in low-sodium versions.

Blackstrap molasses is a very good source of iron, a mineral that is lacking in the Type A Diet. Kelp is an excellent source of iodine and many other minerals. Vinegar should be avoided because the acids tend to cause stomach lining irritation.

Sugar and chocolate are allowed on the Type A Diet, but only in very small amounts. Use them as you would a condiment. Minimize your use of white processed sugar. Recent studies have shown that the immune system is sluggish for several hours after ingesting it.

Highly Beneficial

BARLEY MALT	GARLIC	SOY SAUCE
BLACKSTRAP	GINGER	TAMARI
MOLASSES	MISO	

Neutral

Agar	Corn syrup	Pimiento
Allspice	Cream of tartar	Rice syrup
Almond extract	Cumin	Rosemary
Anise	Curry	Saffron
Arrowroot	Dill	Sage
Basil	Dulse	Salt
Bay leaf	Honey	Savory
Bergamot	Horseradish	Spearmint
Brown rice syrup	Kelp	Sugar, brown
Cardamom	Maple syrup	Sugar, white
Carob	Marjoram	Tamarind
Chervil	Mint	Tapioca
Chives	Mustard (dry)	Tarragon
Chocolate	Nutmeg	Thyme
Cinnamon	Oregano	Turmeric
Cloves	Paprika	Vanilla
Coriander	Parsley	
Cornstarch	Peppermint	

Avoid

Capers	Pepper,	Vinegar, apple cider
Gelatin, plain	peppercorn	Vinegar, balsamic
Pepper, black	Pepper, red	Vinegar, red wine
ground	flakes	Vinegar, white
Pepper, cayenne	Pepper, white	Wintergreen

Condiments

Condiments are not really recommended for any blood type. Type As in particular should avoid products with pickles or vinegar because of their low levels of stomach acid.

Neutral

Jam (from acceptable fruits)	Salad dressing (low-fat, from acceptable ingredients)
Jelly (from acceptable fruits)	
Mustard	

Avoid

Ketchup
Mayonnaise
Pickles
Pickle Relish
Worcestershire sauce

Herbal Teas

The Type A reaction to particular herbal teas is the exact reverse of Type O. While Type Os need to be soothed, Type As need to rev up their immune systems.

Most of your health risk factors as a Type A are related to your sluggish immune system, and certain herbs can have a powerful effect. For example, hawthorn is a cardiovascular tonic; aloe, alfalfa, burdock, and echinacea are immune-system boosters; and green tea possesses important antioxidant effects on the digestive tract, providing protection against cancer.

It is also important for Type As to increase their stomach-acid secretions since they tend to have very low acid levels. Herbs such as ginger and slippery elm increase stomach-acid secretion.

Herbal relaxants, such as chamomile and valerian root, are a perfect fix for stress. The next time you're feeling harried, brew a pot of good tea.

Highly Beneficial

ALFALFA	GINGER	SAINT-JOHN'S-
ALOE	GINSENG	WORT
BURDOCK	GREEN TEA	SLIPPERY ELM
CHAMOMILE	HAWTHORN	STONE ROOT
ECHINACEA	MILK THISTLE	VALERIAN
FENUGREEK	ROSE HIPS	

Neutral

Chickweed	Hops	Peppermint
Coltsfoot	Horehound	Raspberry leaf
Dandelion	Licorice root	Sage
Dong quai	Linden	Sarsaparilla
Elder	Mulberry	Senna
Gentian	Mullein	Shepherd's purse
Goldenseal	Parsley	Skullcap

Spearmint	White birch
Strawberry Leaf	White oak bark
Thyme	Yarrow
Vervain	

Avoid

Catnip	Corn silk	Rhubarb
Cayenne	Red clover	Yellow dock

Miscellaneous Beverages

Red wine is good for Type As because of its positive cardiovascular effects. A glass of red wine every day is believed to lower the risk of heart disease for both men and women.

Coffee may actually be good for Type As. It increases stomach acid and also has the same enzymes found in soy. Alternate coffee and green tea for the best combination of benefits.

All other beverages should be avoided. They don't suit the digestive system of Type As, nor do they support the immune system.

Pure fresh water, of course, should be consumed freely.

Highly Beneficial

COFFEE, DECAF	TEA, GREEN
COFFEE, REGULAR	WINE, RED

Neutral

Wine, white

Avoid

Beer	Soda, cola	Tea, black decaf
Liquor, distilled	Soda, diet	Tea, black regular
Seltzer water	Soda, other	

Meal Planning for Type A

Asterisk (*) indicates the recipe follows.

THE FOLLOWING sample menus and recipes will give you an idea of a typical diet beneficial to Type As. They were developed by Dina Khader, M.S., R.D., a nutritionist who has used the Blood Type Diets successfully with her patients.

These menus are moderate in calories and balanced for metabolic efficiency in Type As. The average person will be able to comfortably maintain weight and even lose weight by following these suggestions. However, alternative food choices are provided if you prefer lighter fare or wish to limit your caloric intake and still eat a balanced, satisfying diet. (The alternative food is listed directly across from the food it replaces.)

Occasionally you will see an ingredient in a recipe that appears on your avoid list. If it is a very small ingredient (such as a dash of spice), you may be able to tolerate it, depending on your condition and whether you are strictly adhering to the diet. However, the meal selections and recipes are generally designed to work very well for Type As.

As you become more familiar with the Type A Diet recommendations, you'll be able to easily create your own menu plans and adjust favorite recipes to make them Type A–friendly.

STANDARD MENU ▪	WEIGHT-CONTROL ALTERNATIVES ▪
SAMPLE MEAL PLAN I	
Breakfast	
water with lemon (on rising)	
oatmeal with soy milk and maple syrup or molasses	cornflakes with soy milk and blueberries

grapefruit juice
coffee or herbal tea

Lunch
Greek salad (chopped lettuce,
    celery, green onions,
    cucumber, with a sprinkling
    of feta cheese, lemon, and
    fresh mint)
apple
1 slice sprouted wheat bread
herbal tea

Midafternoon snack

2 rice cakes with peanut butter	2 rice cakes with honey
2 plums	
green tea or water	

Dinner

*Tofu-Pesto Lasagna	tofu stir-fry with green
broccoli	beans, leeks, snow
frozen yogurt	peas, and alfalfa
coffee or herbal tea	sprouts
(red wine if desired)	

SAMPLE MEAL PLAN 2

Breakfast

water with lemon (on rising)	
*Tofu Omelet	1 poached egg
grapefruit juice	½ cup low-fat yogurt
coffee or herbal tea	with sliced berries

Lunch
miso soup
mixed-green salad
1 slice rye bread
water or herbal tea

Midafternoon snack
*Carob Chip Cookies   *Tofu Dip with raw
or yogurt with fruit   vegetables
herbal tea

Dinner
*Turkey-Tofu Meatballs
steamed zucchini
*String Bean Salad
low-fat frozen yogurt
coffee or herbal tea
(red wine if desired)

S A M P L E   M E A L   P L A N   3

Breakfast
water with lemon (on rising)
*Maple-Walnut Granola with   puffed rice with soy
   soy milk   milk
prune, carrot, or vegetable juice
coffee or herbal tea

Lunch
*Black Bean Soup   cold salmon on salad
mixed-green salad   greens with lemon
                                       juice and olive oil

Midafternoon snack
*Apricot Fruit Bread ½ cup plain yogurt
coffee or herbal tea with drizzle of honey

Dinner
*Arabian Fish Dish *Baked Fish
*Spinach salad
mixed fresh fruit with yogurt
herbal tea
(red wine if desired)

Recipes

TOFU-PESTO LASAGNA

*1 pound soft tofu, mashed with 2 tablespoons olive oil
1 cup shredded part-skim mozzarella cheese
or part-skim ricotta
1 organic egg (optional)
2 packages frozen, chopped spinach or fresh, cut-up spinach
1 teaspoon salt
1 teaspoon oregano
4 cups pesto sauce (you may use less)
9 rice or spelt lasagna noodles, cooked
1 cup water*

Mix tofu and cheese with egg, spinach, and seasonings. Layer 1
cup sauce in 9 x 13-inch baking dish. Layer noodles, then
some of the cheese mixture, then sauce. Repeat, and finish
with noodles and sauce on top.
Bake in oven at 350 degrees F for 30 to 45 minutes or until done.
Makes 4 to 6 servings.

CAROB CHIP COOKIES

⅓ cup organic canola oil
½ cup pure maple syrup
1 teaspoon vanilla extract
1 organic egg
1¾ cups oat or brown rice flour
1 teaspoon baking soda
½ cup carob chips (unsweetened)
dash allspice (optional)

Oil two baking sheets and preheat oven to 375 degrees F. In a medium-size mixing bowl, combine the oil, maple syrup, and vanilla. Beat the egg and stir into the oil mixture. Gradually stir in flour and baking soda to form a stiff batter. Fold in carob chips and drop the batter onto the baking sheets by the teaspoon. Bake for 10 to 15 minutes until cookies are lightly browned. Remove from oven and cool.
Makes 3½ to 4 dozen.

TOFU DIP

1 cup tofu, mashed
1 cup plain nonfat yogurt
1 tablespoon olive oil
juice of 1 lemon
2 tablespoons chopped chives or 1 cup scallions
garlic and salt to season

Combine the tofu, yogurt, olive oil, and lemon juice in a blender and blend at high speed until smooth. Stir in chives or scallions, and seasonings. Remove to a bowl and refrigerate. If mix is too thick to blend well, add a few drops of water.
Serve dip in a glass bowl centered on a platter of fresh vegetables.
Makes approximately 3 cups.

TOFU OMELET

1 pound soft tofu, drained and mashed
5–6 tree oyster mushrooms, sliced
½ pound grated red or white radishes
1 teaspoon mirin or sherry for cooking
1 teaspoon tamari soy sauce
1 tablespoon fresh parsley
1 teaspoon brown rice flour
4 organic eggs, lightly beaten
1 tablespoon canola or extra-virgin olive oil

Combine all the ingredients in a mixing bowl, except for oil. Heat
the oil in a large frying pan. Pour in half the mixture and cover
the pan. Cook over low heat for approximately 15 minutes until egg is cooked. Remove from pan and keep warm.
Repeat the process and use the remainder of the mixture.
Serves 3 to 4.

TURKEY TOFU MEATBALLS

1 pound ground turkey
1 pound container firm tofu
½ cup chestnut flour
1½ cups spelt flour
1 large onion, chopped fine
¼ cup fresh parsley, chopped
2 teaspoons sea salt
4 tablespoons fresh garlic crushed
allowable seasonings to your preference

Mix well. Refrigerate 1 hour. Roll into small meatballs. You can
stir-fry in oil until brown and crisp, or bake in the oven at 350
degrees F for approximately 1 hour.
Makes 4 servings.

STRING BEAN SALAD

1 pound green string beans
juice of 1 lemon
3 tablespoons olive oil
2 cloves garlic, crushed
2 to 3 teaspoons salt

Wash tender, fresh, green string beans. Remove stems and strings.
  Cut into 2-inch pieces.
Cook until tender by boiling in plenty of water. Drain. When cool,
  place in a salad bowl. Dress to taste with lemon juice, olive oil,
  garlic, and salt.
Makes 4 servings.

MAPLE-WALNUT GRANOLA

4 cups rolled oats
1 cup rice bran
1 cup sesame seeds
½ cup dried cranberries
½ cup dried currants
1 cup chopped walnuts
1 teaspoon vanilla extract
¼ cup organic canola oil
¾ cup maple syrup

Preheat oven to 250 degrees F. In a large mixing bowl combine
  the oats, rice bran, seeds, dried fruit, nuts, and vanilla. Add the
  oil and stir evenly.
Pour in maple syrup and mix well until mixture is evenly moistened. Mixture should be crumbly and sticky. Spread mixture
  on a lightly oiled cookie tray and bake for 90 minutes, stirring
  every 15 minutes for even toasting until the mixture is golden
  brown and dry.
Cool thoroughly and store in airtight container.

BLACK BEAN SOUP

1 pound black beans
2 quarts of water
⅛ cup vegetable broth
⅛ pound diced white onion
⅛ pound green onions
¼ pound celery
⅛ pound diced leeks
¼ ounce salt
1 ounce cumin
1 cup dried parsley
1 ounce garlic
1 medium bunch of fresh tarragon (chopped)
1 medium bunch of fresh basil (chopped)
1 medium bunch of scallions

Soak beans in water overnight. Pour off the water and rinse. Add
3 quarts of water and bring beans to a boil.
Discard liquid from the beans and add the vegetable broth. Simmer.
Sauté the onion, celery, leeks, seasonings, and garlic, together in
a pan. Add this mixture to the beans and continue cooking.
Purée ⅛ cup of this soup for consistency. Add scallions at the
end for garnish.
Makes approximately 8 servings.

APRICOT FRUIT BREAD

1¼ cup plain nonfat yogurt
1 organic egg
1 cup apricot conserves (fruit juice sweetened)
2 cups brown rice flour
1 teaspoon ground cinnamon
1 teaspoon ground allspice

1 teaspoon ground nutmeg
1¼ teaspoon baking soda
1 cup chopped, dried, unsulfured apricots
1 cup currants

Grease a standard-size loaf pan and preheat oven to 350 degrees F. In a medium-size bowl, combine the yogurt, egg, and jam. Add 1 cup of flour and half of the spices plus baking soda. Stir until batter is evenly moist.

Add remaining flour and spices. If consistency feels too thick, you can add a few drops of cold water or vanilla soy milk to mixture. Fold in apricots and currants.

Pour batter into greased loaf pan and bake for 40 to 45 minutes until done. Remove bread from the pan and cool on a wire rack.

ARABIAN BAKED FISH

1 large bass or whitefish (3 to 4 pounds)
dash of salt to taste
¼ cup lemon juice
2 tablespoons olive oil
2 large onions, chopped and sautéed in olive oil
2 to 2½ cups tahini sauce (see below)

Wash fish and dry thoroughly. Sprinkle with salt and lemon juice. Let stand for 30 minutes. Drain fish. Place in baking pan after brushing with oil. Bake in a pre-heated oven for 30 minutes at 400 degrees F.

Cover with sautéed onions and tahini sauce, and add a dash of salt. Return to oven and bake until fish is easily flaked with a fork (from 30 to 40 minutes).

Serve the fish on a platter and garnish with parsley and lemon wedges.

Makes 6 to 8 servings.

TAHINI SAUCE

1 cup organic tahini
juice of 3 lemons
2 cloves of garlic, crushed
2 to 3 teaspoons salt
¼ cup dried, organic parsley flakes or fresh parsley,
chopped finely

In a bowl, mix tahini with lemon juice, garlic, salt, and parsley.
Add enough water to make a thick sauce.
Makes approximately 2 cups.

BAKED FISH

1 large whitefish (2 or 3 pounds) or other fish
lemon juice and salt to taste
¼ cup olive oil
1 teaspoon cayenne (optional)
1 teaspoon pepper (optional)
1 teaspoon cumin (optional)

Wash fish. Sprinkle with salt and lemon juice. Add spices if desired. Let stand for ½ hour. Drain.
Coat fish with oil and place in a baking pan. To prevent fish from
drying, wrap with foil, lightly greased with oil. Bake at 350 degrees F in a preheated oven for 30 to 40 minutes, or until fish
is tender and easily flaked.
Makes 4 or 5 servings.

WITH STUFFING (OPTIONAL)

⅓ cup pine nuts or shredded almonds
2 tablespoons olive oil
1 cup parsley, chopped
3 cloves garlic, crushed
salt, pepper, and allspice to taste

Sauté nuts in olive oil until lightly brown. Add parsley and spices and sauté for one minute. Stuff raw fish with the mixture.
Makes 4 to 5 servings.

SPINACH SALAD

2 bunches fresh spinach
1 bunch scallions, chopped
juice of 1 lemon
¼ tablespoon olive oil
salt and pepper to taste (optional)

Wash spinach well. Drain and chop. Sprinkle with salt. After a few minutes, squeeze excess water. Add scallions, lemon juice, oil, salt and pepper. Serve immediately.
Makes 6 servings.

Type A
Supplement Advisory

THE ROLE OF SUPPLEMENTS—be they vitamins, minerals, or herbs—is to add the nutrients that are lacking in your diet or to provide extra protection where you need it. The supplement focus for Type As is:

- Supercharging the immune system
- Supplying cancer-fighting antioxidants
- Preventing infections
- Strengthening the heart

The following recommendations emphasize the supplements that help to meet these goals, and warn against the supplements that can be counterproductive or dangerous for Type As.

Beneficial

VITAMIN B

Type As should be alert to vitamin B-12 deficiency. Not only is the Type A Diet somewhat lacking in this nutrient, which is found mostly in animal proteins, but Type As tend to have a hard time absorbing the B-12 they do eat because they lack intrinsic factor in their stomachs. (Intrinsic factor is a substance produced by the lining of the stomach that helps B-12 be absorbed into the blood.) In elderly Type As, vitamin B-12 deficiency can cause senile dementia and other neurologic impairments.

Most other B vitamins are adequately contained in the Type A Diet. If, however, you suffer from anemia you may want a small supplement of folic acid. Type A heart patients should ask their doctors about low-dose niacin supplements, as niacin has cholesterol-lowering properties.

Best B-Rich Foods for Type As

whole grains (niacin)	tempeh (B-12)
	fish
soy sauce (B-12)	eggs
miso (B-12)	

VITAMIN C

Type As, who have higher rates of stomach cancer because of low stomach acid, can benefit from taking additional supplements of vitamin C. For example, nitrite, a compound that results from the smoking and curing of meats, could be a particular problem with Type As because its cancer-causing potential is greater in people with lower levels of stomach acid. As an antioxidant, vitamin C is known to block this reaction (although you should still avoid smoked and cured foods). However, don't take this to mean that you should take massive amounts. I have found that Type As do not do as well on high doses (1,000 mg and up) of vitamin C because it tends to upset their stomachs. Taken over the course of a day, two to four capsules of a 250 mg supplement, preferably derived from rose hips, should cause no digestive problems.

Best C-Rich Foods for Type As

berries	cherries
grapefruit	lemon
pineapple	broccoli

VITAMIN E

There is some evidence that vitamin E serves as a protectant against both cancer and heart disease—two Type A susceptibilities. You may want to take a daily supplement—no more than 400 IU (international units).

Best E-Rich Foods for Type As

vegetable oil

whole grains

peanuts

leafy green vegetables

CALCIUM

As the Type A diet includes some dairy products, the need for calcium supplementation is not as acute as in Type Os, yet a small amount of additional calcium (300 to 600 mg elemental calcium) from middle age onward is advisable.

In my experience, Type As do better on particular calcium products. The worst source of calcium for Type As is the simplest and most readily available: calcium carbonate (often found in antacids). This form requires the highest amount of stomach acid for absorption. In general, Type As tolerate calcium gluconate, do well on calcium citrate, and do best of all on calcium lactate.

Best Calcium-Rich Foods for Type As

yogurt	canned salmon	broccoli
soy milk	with bones	spinach
eggs	sardines with	
goat milk	bones	

IRON

The Type A Diet is naturally low in iron, which is found in the greatest abundance in red meats. Type A women, especially those with heavy menstrual periods, should be especially careful about keeping sufficient iron stores.

If you need iron supplementation, do it under a doctor's supervision, so blood tests can monitor your progress.

In general, use as low a dose as possible, and avoid extended periods of supplementation. Try to avoid crude iron preparations such as ferrous sulfate, which can irritate your stomach. Milder forms of supplementation, such as iron citrate or blackstrap molasses, may be used instead. Floradix, a liquid iron and herb supplement, can be found at most health food stores and is highly assimilable by Type As.

Best Iron-Rich Foods for Type As

whole grains
beans
figs
blackstrap molasses

ZINC [*with caution*]

I have found that a small amount of zinc supplementation (as little a 3 mg/day) often makes a big difference in protecting children against infections, especially ear infections. Zinc supplementation is a double-edged sword, however. While small, periodic doses enhance immunity, long-term, higher doses depress it and can interfere with the absorption of other minerals. Be careful with zinc! It's completely unregulated and is widely available as a supplement, but you really shouldn't use it without a physician's advice.

Best Zinc-Rich Foods for Type As

eggs
legumes

SELENIUM [*with caution*]
Selenium, which seems to act as a component of the body's own antioxidant defenses, may be of value to cancer-prone Type As. But check with your physician before taking selenium supplements on your own: cases of selenium toxicity have been reported in people who have taken excessive supplements.

CHROMIUM [*with caution*]
Because of a susceptibility to diabetes, Type As with a family history of diabetes may be interested in the fact that chromium enhances the effectiveness of the body's glucose-tolerance factor, which increases the efficiency of insulin. However, we know very little about the long-term effects of chromium supplementation, and I would not advise using it at this time. Type As can best protect themselves from diabetic complications by following the blood type diet.

Herbs/Phytochemicals
Recommended for Type As

HAWTHORN *(Crataegus oxyacantha)*. Hawthorn is a great cardiovascular tonic. Type As should definitely add it to their diet regimen if they or members of their family have a history of heart disease. This phytochemical, with exceptional preventive capacities, is found in the Hawthorn tree *(Crataegus oxyacantha)*. It has a number of impressive cardiovascular effects. Hawthorn increases the elasticity of the arteries and strengthens the heart, while also lowering blood pressure and exerting a mild solvent-like effect upon the plaques in the arteries.

Officially approved for pharmaceutical use in Germany, the actions of hawthorn are virtually unknown elsewhere. Extracts and tinctures are readily available through naturopathic physicians, health food stores, and pharmacies. I cannot praise this herb too highly. Official German government monographs show the plant to be completely free of any side effects. If I had my way, extracts of hawthorn would be used to fortify breakfast cereals, just as vitamins are.

IMMUNE-ENHANCING HERBS. Because the immune systems of Type As tend to be open to immune-compromising infections, gentle immune-enhancing herbs, such as purple coneflower *(Echinacea purpurea)*, can help ward off colds or flus and may help optimize the immune system's anti-cancer surveillance. Many people take echinacea in liquid or tablet form. It is widely available. The Chinese herb huangki *(Astragalus membranaceous)* is also taken as an immune tonic, but is not as easy to find. In both herbs the active principles are sugars that act as mitogens that stimulate proliferation of white blood cells which act in defense of the immune systems.

CALMING HERBS. Type As can use mild herbal relaxants, such as chamomile and valerian root, as an anti-stress factor. These herbs are available as teas and should be taken frequently. Valerian has a bit of a pungent odor, which actually becomes pleasing once you get used to it. There is a rumor sometimes heard in health food stores that valerian is the natural form of Valium (diazepam), a prescription tranquilizer. This is wrong. Valerian was named for a Roman emperor who had the misfortune to be captured in battle by the Persians. Killed, stuffed, dyed red, and exhibited in a Persian museum, Valerian is fortunate to have had anything named for him.

QUERCETIN. Quercetin is a bioflavonoid found abundantly in vegetables, particularly yellow onions. Quercetin supplements are widely available in health food stores, usually in capsules of 100 to 500 mg. Quercetin is a very powerful antioxidant, many hundreds of times more potent than vitamin E. It can make a powerful addition to Type A cancer-prevention strategies.

MILK THISTLE *(Silybum marianum)*. Like quercetin, milk thistle is an effective antioxidant with the additional special property of reaching very high concentrations in the liver and bile ducts. Type As can suffer from disorders of the liver and gallbladder. If your family has any history of liver, pancreas, or gallbladder problems, consider adding a milk thistle supplement (easily found in most health food stores) to your protocol. Cancer patients who are receiving chemotherapy should use a milk thistle supplement to help protect their livers from damage.

BROMELAIN (pineapple enzymes). If you are Type A and suffer from bloating or other signs of poor absorption of protein, take a bromelain supplement. This enzyme has a moderate ability to break down dietary proteins, helping the Type A digestive tract assimilate proteins better.

PRO-BIOTIC SUPPLEMENTS. If the Type A Diet is new for you, you may find that adjusting to a vegetarian diet is uncomfortable and produces excessive gas or bloating. A pro-biotic supplement can counter this effect by supplying the "good" bacteria usually found in the digestive tract. Look for pro-biotic supplements high in "bifidus factor," as this strain of bacteria is best suited to the Type A system.

Avoid

VITAMIN A–BETA CAROTENE
My father always avoided giving beta carotene to his Type A patients, saying that it irritated their blood vessels. I questioned his

observation, as it had never been documented. Quite to the contrary, the evidence suggested that beta carotene may prevent artery disease. Yet recently there have been studies suggesting that beta carotene in high doses may act as a pro-oxidant, speeding up damage to the tissues rather than stopping it. Perhaps my father's observation was correct, at least in the case of Type As. If this is so, perhaps Type As may wish to forgo beta carotene supplements and consume high levels of carotenoids in their diet instead.

One caveat: As we age, our ability to assimilate the fat-soluble vitamins may diminish. Elderly Type As might benefit from small supplemental doses of vitamin A (10,000 IU daily) to help counteract the effects of aging upon the immune system.

Best Carotene-Rich Foods for Type As

eggs	spinach
yellow squash	broccoli
carrots	

Type A Stress/Exercise Profile

THE ABILITY to reverse the negative effects of stress lives in your blood type. As we discussed in chapter 3, stress is not in itself a problem; it's how you respond to stress. Each blood type has a distinct, genetically programmed instinct for overcoming stress.

Type As react to the first stage of stress—the alarm stage—intellectually. Adrenergically charged bulbs flash in your brain, producing anxiety, irritability, and hyperactivity. As the stress signals throb in your immune system, you grow weaker. The heightened sensitivity of your nervous system gradually frays your delicate protective antibodies. You're too weary to fight the infections and bacteria that are waiting to jump in like muggers trailing an intoxicated prey.

If, however, you adopt quieting techniques, such as yoga or meditation, you can achieve great benefits by countering negative stresses with focus and relaxation. Type As do not respond well to continuous confrontation, and need to consider and practice the art of stillness as a calming charm.

If Type As remain in their naturally tense state, stress can produce heart disease and various forms of cancer. Exercises that provide calm and focus are the remedy that pull the Type A from the grip of stress.

Tai chi chuan, the slow-motion, ritualistic pattern of Chinese boxing, and hatha yoga, the timeless Indian stretching system, are calming, centering experiences. Moderate isotonic exercises, such as hiking, swimming, and bicycling, are favored for Type As. When I advise calming exercises, it doesn't mean you can't break a sweat. The key is really your mental engagement in your physical activity.

For example, heavy competitive sports and exercises will only exhaust your nervous energy, make you tense all over again, and leave your immune system open to illness or disease.

The following exercises are recommended for Type As. Pay special attention to the length of the sessions. To achieve a consistent release of tension and revival of energy, you need to perform one or more of these exercises three or four times a week.

EXERCISE	DURATION	FREQUENCY
TAI CHI	30–45 min.	3–5x week
HATHA YOGA	30 min.	3–5x week
MARTIAL ARTS	60 min.	2–3x week
GOLF	60 min.	2–3x week
BRISK WALKING	20–40 min.	2–3x week
SWIMMING	30 min.	3–4x week
DANCE	30–45 min.	2–3x week
AEROBICS (LOW IMPACT)	30–45 min.	2–3x week
STRETCHING	15 min.	3–5x week

Type A Exercise Guidelines

TAI CHI CHUAN, or tai chi, is an exercise that enhances the flexibility of body movement. The slow, graceful, elegant gestures of tai chi chuan routines seem to mask the full-speed hand and foot blows, blocks, and parries they represent. In China, tai chi is practiced daily by groups who gather in public squares to perform the movements in unison. Tai chi can be a very effective relaxation technique, although it takes concentration and patience to master.

Yoga is also good for the Type A stress pattern. It combines inner rectitude with breath control and postures designed to allow for complete concentration without distraction by worldly concerns. Hatha yoga is the most common form of yoga practiced in the West.

If you learn basic yoga postures, you can create a routine best suited to your lifestyle. Many Type As who have adopted yoga relaxation tell me that they will not leave the house until they do their yoga.

However, some patients have told me that they are concerned that adopting yoga practices may conflict with their religious beliefs. They fear that the practice of yoga implies that they have adopted Eastern mysticism. I respond, "If you eat Italian food, does that make you Italian?" Meditation and yoga are what you make of them. Visualize and meditate on those subjects that are relevant to you. The postures are neutral; they are just timeless and proven movements.

SIMPLE YOGA RELAXATION TECHNIQUES

Yoga begins and ends with relaxation. We contract our muscles constantly, but rarely do we think of doing the opposite—letting go and relaxing. We can feel better and be healthier if we regularly release the tensions left behind within the muscles by the stresses and strains of life.

The best position for relaxation is lying on your back. Arrange your arms and legs so that you are completely comfortable in your hips, shoulders, and back. The goal of deep relaxation is to let your body and mind settle down to soothing calmness, in the same way that an agitated pool of water eventually calms to stillness.

Begin with abdominal breathing. As a baby breathes, its abdomen moves, not its chest. However, many of us grow to unconsciously adopt the unnatural and inefficient habit of restrained chest breathing. One of the aims of yoga is to make you aware of the true center of breathing. Observe the pattern of your breathing. Is your breathing fast, shallow, and irregular, or do you tend to hold your breath? Allow your breathing to revert to a more natural pattern—full, deep, regular, and with no constriction. Try to isolate just your lower breathing muscles; see if you can breathe without moving your chest. Breathing exercises are always done smoothly and without any strain. Place one hand on your navel and feel the movement of your breathing. Relax your shoulders.

Start the exercise by breathing out completely. When you inhale, pretend that a heavy weight, such as a large book, is resting on your navel, and that by your inhalation, you are trying to raise this imaginary weight up toward the ceiling.

Then, when you exhale, simply let this imaginary weight press down against your abdomen, helping you to exhale. Exhale more air out than you normally would, as if to "squeeze" more air out of your lungs. This will act as a yoga stretch for the diaphragm and further help release tension in this muscle. Bring your abdominal muscles into play here to assist. When you inhale, direct your breath down so deeply that you are lifting an imaginary heavy weight up toward the ceiling. Try to completely coordinate and isolate the abdominal breath with no chest or rib movement.

Even if you perform more aerobic exercises during the course of your week, try to integrate the relaxing, soothing routines that will help you best manage your Type A stress patterns.

A Final Note:
The Personality Question

BLOOD TYPE A was originally adapted to deal with dense population concentrations and the stresses of a more sedentary but intense urban lifestyle. Certain psychological traits would develop in people who must tolerate the demands of a crowded environment.

Probably the most important quality a person must have in that setting is a cooperative nature. The original Type As had to be decent, orderly, and law abiding, and had to exhibit self-control. Communities can't exist if there is no respect for others and their property. Loners do poorly in group settings. If the characteristics of Type Os had not evolved to suit an agrarian society, the result would have been chaos—and ultimately doom. Again, it's thanks to our Type A ancestors that humans survived.

The early Type As had to be clever, sensitive, passionate, and very smart to meet the challenges of a more complex life. But all of these qualities had to exist within a framework. That may be the reason why Type As, even today, tend to have more tightly wired systems. They bottle up their anxiety—because that's what you do when you're trying to get along with others—but when they explode, watch out! The antidotes to this tremendous inner stress are, as we have discussed, the more soothing and contemplative relaxation exercises of yoga and tai chi chuan.

It would seem that Type As are poorly suited for the intense, highly pressured leadership positions at which Type Os excel. That's not to say they can't be leaders. But they instinctively reject the dog-eat-dog manner of contemporary leadership. When Type As get into these positions, they tend to unravel. Former American presidents Lyndon B. Johnson, Richard Nixon, and Jimmy Carter were all Type A. While each man brought an unquestioned brilliance and passion to the job, all of them possessed fatal flaws. When the stress got too great, they became anxious and paranoid, taking everything personally. In the end, it was these Type A responses that forced each of them out of office.

Perhaps the most notorious Type A was Adolf Hitler. While most people might associate him with the sheer drive and brutal surety of the Type O leader, Hitler's overriding trait was really an extraordinary hypersensitivity that led him ultimately to madness. Hitler was an anomalous being. His obsession with a genetically ordered society was that of a mutated Type A personality with a nightmarish vision.

Blood Type

B

Plan

TYPE B: *The Nomad*

- BALANCED
- STRONG IMMUNE SYSTEM
- TOLERANT DIGESTIVE SYSTEM
- MOST FLEXIBLE DIETARY CHOICES
- DAIRY EATER
- RESPONDS BEST TO STRESS
  WITH CREATIVITY
- REQUIRES A BALANCE BETWEEN PHYSICAL
  AND MENTAL ACTIVITY TO STAY LEAN
  AND SHARP.

The Type B Diet

TYPE O AND TYPE A seem to be polar opposites in many respects. But Type B can best be described as idiosyncratic—with utterly unique and sometimes chameleonlike characteristics. In many respects, Type B resembles Type O so much that the two seem related. Then, suddenly, Type B will take on a totally unfamiliar shape—one that is peculiarly its own. You might say that Type B represents a sophisticated refinement in the evolutionary journey, an effort to join together divergent peoples and cultures.

On the whole, the sturdy and alert Type Bs are usually able to resist many of the most severe diseases common to modern life, such as heart disease and cancer. Even when they do contract these diseases, they are more likely to survive them. Yet because Type Bs are somewhat offbeat, their systems seem more prone to exotic immune-system disorders, such as multiple sclerosis, lupus, and chronic fatigue syndrome (see chapter 9).

In my experience, a Type B who carefully follows the recommended diet can often bypass severe disease and live a long and healthy life.

The Type B Diet is balanced and wholesome, including a wide variety of foods. In the words of my father, it represents "the best of the animal and vegetable kingdoms." Think of B as standing for balance—the balancing forces of A and O.

The Weight-Loss Factor

FOR TYPE BS, the biggest factors in weight gain are corn, buckwheat, lentils, peanuts, and sesame seeds. Each of these foods has a different lectin, but all of them affect the efficiency of your metabolic process, resulting in fatigue, fluid retention, and hypoglycemia—a severe drop in blood sugar after eating a meal. My patients with hypoglycemia often ask me if they should follow the standard advice of eating several small meals a day in order to keep their blood sugar levels from dropping. I discourage this practice. I find that the major problem is not when they eat, but what they eat. Certain foods trigger a drop in blood sugar—especially for Type Bs. When you eliminate these foods and begin eating the right diet for your type, your blood sugar levels should remain normal after meals. The problem with "grazing"—eating many small meals throughout the day—is that it interferes with your body's natural hunger signals; you may begin to find that you are hungry all the time—not a very helpful situation if you're trying to lose weight.

Type Bs are similar to Type Os in their reaction to the gluten found in wheat germ and whole wheat products. The gluten lectin adds to the problems caused by the other metabolism-slowing foods. When food is not efficiently digested and burned as fuel for the body, it gets stored as fat.

In itself, the wheat gluten doesn't attack Type Bs as severely as it does Type Os. However, when you add wheat to the mix of corn, lentils, buckwheat, and peanuts, the end result is just as damaging. Type Bs who want to lose weight should definitely avoid wheat.

When these foods are avoided, along with others that contain toxic lectins, it has been my experience that Type Bs are very successful in controlling their weight. You don't have any natural physiological barriers to weight loss, such as the thyroid problems that can hamper Type Os. Nor do you suffer from digestive disorders. All you need to do to lose weight is stay on your diet.

Some people are surprised that Type Bs aren't more likely to have problems with weight control, since dairy foods are encouraged on their diet. Of course, if you overeat high-calorie foods, you're going to gain weight! But the moderate consumption of dairy foods actually helps Type Bs achieve a metabolic balance. The real culprits are the particular foods that inhibit the efficient use of energy and promote the storage of calories as fat.

These are the highlights for Type B weight loss:

FOODS THAT ENCOURAGE WEIGHT GAIN

CORN	*inhibits insulin efficiency*
	hampers metabolic rate
	causes hypoglycemia
LENTILS	*inhibit proper nutrient uptake*
	hamper metabolic efficiency
	cause hypoglycemia
PEANUTS	*hamper metabolic efficiency*
	cause hypoglycemia
	inhibit liver function
SESAME SEEDS	*hamper metabolic efficiency*
	cause hypoglycemia
BUCKWHEAT	*inhibits digestion*
	hampers metabolic efficiency
	causes hypoglycemia
WHEAT	*slows the digestive and metabolic processes*
	causes food to be stored as fat, not burned as energy
	inhibits insulin eficiency

FOODS THAT ENCOURAGE WEIGHT LOSS

GREEN VEGETABLES	*aid efficient metabolism*
MEAT	*aids efficient metabolism*
LIVER	*aids efficient metabolism*
EGGS/LOW-FAT DAIRY PRODUCTS	*aid efficient metabolism*
LICORICE TEA*	*counters hypoglycemia*

*Never take licorice supplements without a doctor's supervision. Licorice tea is okay.

INCORPORATE THESE GUIDELINES INTO THE TOTAL PICTURE OF THE TYPE B DIET, WHICH FOLLOWS.

Meats and Poultry

BLOOD TYPE B	WEEKLY ▪ IF YOUR ANCESTRY IS			
Food	Portion*	African	Caucasian	Asian
LEAN RED MEATS	4–6 OZ. *(men)* 2–5 OZ. *(women and children)*	3–4X	2–3X	2–3X
POULTRY	4–6 OZ. *(men)* 2–5 OZ. *(women and children)*	0–2X	0–3X	0–2X

The portion recommendations are merely guidelines that can help refine your diet according to ancestral propensities.

There appears to be a direct connection between stress, autoimmune disorders, and red meat in the Type B system. That's because your Type B ancestors adapted better to other kinds of meats. (After all, there weren't a lot of steer on the Siberian tundra!) If you are fatigued or suffer from immune deficiencies, you should eat red meat such as lamb, mutton, or rabbit several times a week, in preference to beef or turkey.

In my experience, one of the most difficult adjustments Type Bs must make is giving up chicken. Chicken contains a Blood Type B agglutinating lectin in its muscle tissue. If you're accustomed to eating more poultry than red meat, you can eat other poultry such as turkey or pheasant. Although they are similar to chicken in many respects, neither contains the dangerous lectin.

The news about chicken is troubling to many people because it has become a fundamental part of many ethnic diets. In addition, people have been told to eat chicken instead of beef because it is "healthier." But here is another case where one dietary guideline does not fit all. Chicken may be leaner (although not always) than red meat, but that isn't the issue. The issue is the power of an agglutinating lectin to attack your bloodstream and potentially lead to strokes and immune disorders. So, even though chicken may be a beloved food, I urge you to begin weaning yourself away from it.

Highly Beneficial

LAMB	RABBIT
MUTTON	VENISON

Neutral

Beef	Pheasant
Beef, ground	Turkey
Buffalo	Veal
Liver	

Avoid

Bacon	Goose	Pork
Chicken	Ham	Quail
Cornish hens	Heart	
Duck	Partridge	

Seafood

BLOOD TYPE B		WEEKLY ■ IF YOUR ANCESTRY IS		
Food	*Portion*	*African*	*Caucasian*	*Asian*
ALL RECOMMENDED SEAFOOD	4–6 OZ.	4–6x	3–5x	3–5x

Type Bs thrive on seafood, especially deep-ocean fish such as cod and salmon, which are rich in nutritious oils. White fish, such as flounder, halibut, and sole, are also excellent sources of high-quality protein for Type Bs. Avoid all shellfish—crab, lobster, shrimp, mussels, etc. They contain lectins that are disruptive to the Type B system. It is interesting to note that many of the original Type Bs were Jewish tribes that forbade the consumption of shellfish. Perhaps this dietary law was an acknowledgment that shellfish are poorly digested by Type Bs.

Highly Beneficial

COD	MAHIMAHI	SEA TROUT
FLOUNDER	MONKFISH	SHAD
GROUPER	OCEAN PERCH	SOLE
HADDOCK	PICKEREL	STURGEON
HAKE	PIKE	STURGEON
HALIBUT	PORGY	EGGS (CAVIAR)
MACKEREL	SARDINE	

Neutral

Abalone	Red snapper	Squid (calamari)
Albacore (tuna)	Sailfish	Swordfish
Bluefish	Salmon	Tilefish
Carp	Scallop	Weakfish
Catfish	Shark	White perch
Herring (fresh)	Silver Perch	Whitefish
Herring (pickled)	Smelt	Yellow perch
Rainbow trout	Snapper	

Avoid

Anchovy	Eel	Sea bass
Barracuda	Frog	Shrimp
Beluga	Lobster	Snail
Bluegill bass	Lox (smoked	Striped bass
Clam	salmon)	Turtle
Conch	Mussels	Yellowtail
Crab	Octopus	
Crayfish	Oysters	

Dairy and Eggs

BLOOD TYPE B		WEEKLY • IF YOUR ANCESTRY IS		
Food	Portion	African	Caucasian	Asian
EGGS	I EGG	3–4X	3–4X	5–6X
CHEESES	2 OZ.	3–4X	3–5X	2–3X
YOGURT	4–6 OZ.	0–4X	2–4X	1–3X
MILK	4–6 OUNCES	0–3X	4–5X	2–3X

Type B is the only blood type that can fully enjoy a variety of dairy foods. That's because the primary sugar in the Type B antigen is D-galactosamine, the very same sugar present in milk. Dairy foods were first introduced to the human diet during the height of the Type B development, along with the domestication of animals. (By the way, eggs do not contain the lectin that is found in the muscle tissues of chicken.)

However, there are ancestral idiosyncrasies that blur the picture. If you are of Asian descent, you may initially have a problem adapting to dairy foods—not because your system is resistant to them, but because your culture typically has been resistant. Dairy products were first introduced into Asian societies with the invasion of the Mongolian hordes. To the Asian mind, dairy products were the food of the barbarian, and thus not fit to eat. The stigma remains to this day, although there are large numbers of Type Bs in Asia whose soy-based diet is damaging to their systems.

Type Bs of African descent might also have trouble adapting to dairy foods. Type Bs are barely represented in Africa, and many Africans are lactose intolerant.

These intolerances should not be confused with allergies. Allergies are immune responses that cause your blood to produce an antibody to the food. Intolerances are digestive problems you may have with certain foods. Intolerances are caused by migration, cultural assimilation, and other factors—for example, when Type Bs moved into Africa, where dairy foods were not prominent.

What can you do? If you are lactose intolerant, begin using a lactase enzyme preparation, which will make digestion of dairy foods possible. Then, after you have been on your Type B Diet for several weeks, slowly introduce dairy foods, beginning with cultured or soured dairy products, such as yogurt and kefir, which may be tolerated better than fresh milk products, such as ice cream, whole milk, and cream cheese. I've found that lactose-intolerant Type Bs often are able to incorporate dairy foods after they have corrected the overall problems in their diets.

Soy foods often are recommended as dairy substitutes. You may eat soy foods, but they're mostly benign for Type Bs. They don't have the many health benefits for you that they have for Type As. Part of my concern about recommending soy for Type Bs is the danger that people will often substitute them as main courses, instead of eating the meat, fish, and dairy that Type Bs really need for optimum health.

Highly Beneficial

COTTAGE	KEFIR	YOGURT WITH
CHEESE	MOZZARELLA	FRUIT
FARMER	RICOTTA	YOGURT,
FETA	SKIM OR 2%	FROZEN
GOAT CHEESE	MILK	
GOAT MILK	YOGURT	

Neutral

Brie	Cheddar	Gouda
Butter	Colby	Gruyère
Buttermilk	Cream cheese	Jarlsberg
Camembert	Edam	Monterey jack
Casein	Emmenthal	Munster

Neufchatel	Sherbet	Swiss
Parmesan	Soy cheese	Whey
Provolone	Soy milk	Whole milk

Avoid

American cheese	Ice cream
Blue cheese	String cheese

Oils and Fats

BLOOD TYPE B		WEEKLY ▪ IF YOUR ANCESTRY IS		
Food	*Portion*	*African*	*Caucasian*	*Asian*
OILS	I TABLESPOON	3–5X	4–6X	5–7X

Introduce olive oil into your diet to encourage proper digestion and healthy elimination. Use at least one tablespoon every other day. Ghee, an Indian preparation of clarified butter, also can be used in cooking. Avoid sesame, sunflower, and corn oils, which contain lectins that are damaging to the Type B digestive tract.

Highly Beneficial

OLIVE OIL

Neutral

Cod liver oil
Linseed (flaxseed) oil

Avoid

Canola oil	Safflower oil
Corn oil	Sesame oil
Cottonseed oil	Sunflower oil
Peanut oil	

Nuts and Seeds

BLOOD TYPE B		WEEKLY ▪ IF YOUR ANCESTRY IS		
Food	*Portion*	*African*	*Caucasian*	*Asian*
NUTS AND SEEDS	6–8 NUTS	3–5X	2–5X	2–3X
NUT BUTTERS	I TABLESPOON	2–3X	2–3X	2–3X

Most nuts and seeds are not advised for Type Bs. Peanuts, sesame seeds, and sunflower seeds, among others, contain lectins that interfere with Type B insulin production.

It might be difficult for Type B Asians to give up sesame seeds and sesame-based products, but in this case, your blood type speaks more definitively than your culture.

Neutral

Almond butter   Nuts, chestnuts   Nuts, macadamia
Nuts, almonds   Nuts, hickory   Nuts, pecans
Nuts, Brazil nuts   Nuts, litchi   Nuts, walnuts

Avoid

Nuts, cashews   Peanut butter   Sunflower butter
Nuts, filberts   Poppy seeds   Sunflower seeds
Nuts, pignola   Pumpkin seeds
  (pine)   Sesame butter
Nuts, pistachio   (tahini)
Peanuts   Sesame seeds

Beans and Legumes

BLOOD TYPE B		WEEKLY ■ IF YOUR ANCESTRY IS		
Food	*Portion*	*African*	*Caucasian*	*Asian*
ALL RECOMMENDED BEANS AND LEGUMES	1 CUP, DRY	3–4X	2–3X	4–5X

Type Bs can eat some beans and legumes, but many beans, such as lentils, garbanzos, pintos, and black-eyed peas, contain lectins that interfere with the production of insulin.

Generally, Type B Asians tolerate beans and legumes better than do other Type Bs because they are culturally accustomed to them. But even Asians should limit their selection of these foods to those that are highly beneficial, and eat them sparingly.

Highly Beneficial

BEANS, KIDNEY   BEANS, NAVY
BEANS, LIMA

Neutral

Beans, broad	Beans, jicama	Beans, string
Beans, cannellini	Beans, northern	Beans, tamarind
Beans, copper	Beans, red	Beans, white
Beans, fava	Beans, snap	Peas, green
Beans, green	Beans, soy	Peas, pods

Avoid

Beans, aduke	Beans, garbanzo	Lentils, green
Beans, azuki	Beans, pinto	Lentils, red
Beans, black	Lentils, domestic	Peas, black-eyed

Cereals

BLOOD TYPE B		WEEKLY ■ IF YOUR ANCESTRY IS		
Food	*Portion*	*African*	*Caucasian*	*Asian*
ALL CEREALS	I CUP, DRY	2–3X	2–4X	2–4X

When Type B is in good balance—that is, following the fundamental tenets of the diet—wheat may not be a problem. However, wheat is not tolerated well by most Type Bs. Wheat contains a lectin that attaches to the insulin receptors in the fat cells, prohibiting insulin from attaching. The result is reduced insulin efficiency and failure to stimulate fat "burning."

Type Bs also should avoid rye, which contains a lectin that settles in the vascular system, causing blood disorders and potentially strokes. (It is interesting to note that the main victims of vascular disease, sometimes called St. Anthony's fire, are the largely Type B population of eastern European Jews. Rye bread is a popular part of their cultural tradition.)

Corn and buckwheat are major factors in Type B weight gain. More than any other food, they contribute to a sluggish metabolism, insulin irregularity, fluid retention, and fatigue.

Again, for Type Bs the key is balance. Eat a variety of grains and cereals. Rice and oats are excellent choices. I also urge you to try spelt, which is highly beneficial for Type Bs.

Highly Beneficial

MILLET	OATMEAL	RICE BRAN
OAT BRAN	RICE, PUFFED	SPELT

Neutral

Cream of rice	Granola
Familia	Grape nuts
Farina	

Avoid

Amaranth	Cream of wheat	Shredded wheat
Barley	Kamut	Wheat bran
Buckwheat	Kasha	Wheat germ
Cornflakes	Rye	
Cornmeal	Seven-grain	

Breads and Muffins

BLOOD TYPE B		DAILY ▪ IF YOUR ANCESTRY IS		
Food	*Portion*	*African*	*Caucasian*	*Asian*
BREADS, CRACKERS	1 SLICE	0–1X	0–1X	0–1X
MUFFINS	1 MED. MUFFIN	0–1X	0–1X	0–1X

The recommendations here are similar to those for cereals. Avoid wheat, corn, buckwheat, and rye. That still leaves you a wide variety of breads to choose from. Try Essene or Ezekiel bread, found in health food stores. These "live" breads are highly nutritious. Although they are sprouted wheat breads, the problem kernel is destroyed in the sprouting process, and they are perfectly healthful.

Highly Beneficial

BROWN RICE BREAD	EZEKIEL BREAD	RICE CAKES
	FIN CRISP	WASA BREAD
ESSENE BREAD	MILLET	

Neutral

Gluten-free bread	Ideal Flat Bread	Spelt bread
High-protein no-wheat bread	Oat bran muffins	Soy flour bread
	Pumpernickel	

Avoid

Bagels, wheat	100% rye bread	Whole wheat
Corn muffins	Rye Crisp	bread
Durum wheat	Rye Vita	
Multi-grain bread	Wheat bran muffins	

Grains and Pasta

BLOOD TYPE B		WEEKLY ■ IF YOUR ANCESTRY IS		
Food	*Portion*	*African*	*Caucasian*	*Asian*
GRAINS	I CUP, DRY	3–4X	3–4X	2–3X
PASTAS	I CUP, DRY	3–4X	3–4X	2–3X

The Type B grain and pasta choices are absolutely consistent with the cereal and bread recommendations. I would, however, advise that you moderate your intake of pasta and rice. You won't need many of these nutrients if you're consuming the meat, seafood, and dairy products advised.

Highly Beneficial

FLOUR, OAT
FLOUR, RICE

Neutral

Flour, Graham	Pasta, semolina	Rice, basmati
Flour, spelt	Pasta, spinach	Rice, brown
Flour, white	Quinoa	Rice, white

Avoid

Buckwheat	Couscous	Flour, bulgur
kasha	Flour, barley	wheat

Flour, Durum wheat	Flour, rye	Pasta, artichoke
Flour, gluten	Flour, whole wheat	Noodles, soba
		Rice, wild

Vegetables

BLOOD TYPE B	DAILY ▪ ALL ANCESTRAL TYPES	
Food	*Portion*	
RAW	I CUP, PREPARED	3–5X
COOKED	I CUP, PREPARED	3–5X

There are many high-quality, nutritious, Type B–friendly vegetables—so take full advantage with three to five servings a day. There is only a handful of vegetables that Type Bs should avoid, but take these guidelines to heart.

Eliminate tomatoes completely from your diet. The tomato is a rare vegetable called a panhemaglutinan. That means it contains lectins that can agglutinate every blood type. While the tomato lectin has little effect on Type O or Type AB, both Type B and Type A suffer strong reactions, usually in the form of irritations of the stomach lining.

Corn is also off your list, as it contains those insulin- and metabolism-upsetting lectins mentioned before. Also avoid olives, since their molds can trigger allergic reactions.

Since Type Bs tend to be more vulnerable to viruses and autoimmune diseases, eat plenty of leafy green vegetables, which contain magnesium, an important antiviral agent. Magnesium also is helpful for Type B children who have eczema.

For the most part, the vegetable world is your kingdom. Unlike other blood types, you can fully enjoy potatoes and yams, cabbages and mushrooms—and many other delicious foods from nature's bounty.

Highly Beneficial

BEETS
BEET LEAVES
BROCCOLI
CABBAGE,
    CHINESE
CABBAGE, RED
CABBAGE,
    WHITE
CARROTS
CAULIFLOWER
COLLARD
    GREENS
EGGPLANT

KALE
LIMA BEANS
MUSHROOM,
    SHIITAKE
MUSTARD
    GREENS
PARSLEY
PARSNIPS
PEPPERS,
    GREEN
PEPPERS,
    JALAPEÑO
PEPPERS, RED

PEPPERS,
    YELLOW
POTATOES,
    SWEET
SPROUTS,
    BRUSSELS
YAMS, ALL
    TYPES

Neutral

Arugula
Asparagus
Bamboo shoots
Bok choy
Celery
Chervil
Chicory
Cucumber
Daikon radish
Dandelion
Dill
Endive
Escarole
Fennel
Fiddlehead ferns
Garlic
Ginger
Horseradish
Kohlrabi

Leek
Lettuce, Bibb
Lettuce, Boston
Lettuce, iceberg
Lettuce, romaine
Lettuce, mesclun
Mushroom,
    abalone
Mushroom,
    domestic
Mushroom, enoki
Mushroom,
    Portobello
Mushroom,
    tree oyster
Okra
Onions, green
Onions, red
Onions, Spanish

Onions, yellow
Potatoes, red
Potatoes, white
Radicchio
Rappini
Rutabaga
Scallion
Seaweed
Shallots
Snow peas
Spinach
Sprouts, alfalfa
Squash, all types
Swiss chard
Turnips
Water chestnut
Watercress
Zucchini

Avoid

Artichoke, domestic	Corn, yellow	Radishes
Artichoke, Jerusalem	Olives, black	Sprouts, mung
	Olives, green	Sprouts, radish
Avocado	Olives, Greek	Tempeh
Corn, white	Olives, Spanish	Tofu
	Pumpkin	Tomato

Fruits

BLOOD TYPE B	DAILY ▪ ALL ANCESTRAL TYPES	
Food	*Portion*	
ALL RECOMMENDED FRUITS	I FRUIT OR 3–5 OZ.	3–4X

You'll notice that there are very few fruits a Type B must avoid—and they're pretty uncommon in any case. Most Type Bs won't sorely miss persimmons, pomegranates, or prickly pears in their diets.

Pineapple can be particularly good for Type Bs who are susceptible to bloating—especially if you're not used to eating the dairy foods and meats on your diet. Bromelain, an enzyme in the pineapple, helps you digest your food more easily.

On the whole, you can choose your fruits liberally from the following lists. Type Bs tend to have very balanced digestive systems, with a healthy acid-alkaline level, so you may have some of the fruits that are too acidic for other blood types.

Try to incorporate at least one or two fruits from the highly beneficial list every day to take advantage of their pro-B medicinal qualities.

Highly Beneficial

BANANAS	GRAPES, GREEN	PLUMS, GREEN
CRANBERRIES	GRAPES, RED	PLUMS, RED
GRAPES, BLACK	PAPAYA	
GRAPES, CONCORD	PINEAPPLE	
	PLUMS, DARK	

Neutral

Apples	Guava	Melon, Spanish
Apricots	Kiwi	Melon, watermelon
Blackberries	Kumquat	Nectarines
Blueberries	Lemons	Oranges
Boysenberries	Limes	Peaches
Cherries	Loganberries	Pears
Currants, black	Mangoes	Plantains
Currants, red	Melon, canang	Prunes
Dates	Melon, cantaloupe	Raisins
Elderberries	Melon, casaba	Raspberries
Figs, dried	Melon, Christmas	Strawberries
Figs, fresh	Melon, Crenshaw	Tangerines
Gooseberries	Melon, honeydew	
Grapefruit	Melon, musk	

Avoid

Coconuts	Rhubarb
Persimmons	Starfruit
Pomegranates	(carambola)
Prickly pear	

Juices and Fluids

BLOOD TYPE B	DAILY ■ ALL ANCESTRAL TYPES	
Food	*Portion*	
ALL RECOMMENDED JUICES	8 OZ.	2–3X
WATER	8 OZ.	4–7X

Most fruit and vegetable juices are okay for Type Bs. If you'd like a daily juice with built-in immune- and nervous-system boosters designed for Type Bs, try the following beverage first thing every morning. I call it the Membrane Fluidizer Cocktail, but I assure you that it's much more alluring than its name implies.

Mix 1 tablespoon of flaxseed oil, 1 tablespoon of high-quality lecithin granules, and 6 to 8 ounces of fruit juice. Shake and drink. Lecithin is an lipid, found in animals and plants, that contains metabolism- and immune system–enhancing properties. You can find lecithin granules in your local health food store and in some supermarkets.

The Membrane Fluidizer Cocktail provides high levels of choline, serine, and ethanolamine (the phospholipids), which are of great value to Type Bs. You may be surprised to find that it's rather tasty, because the lecithin emulsifies the oil, allowing it to mix with the juice.

Highly Beneficial

CABBAGE	PAPAYA
CRANBERRY	PINEAPPLE
GRAPE	

Neutral

Apple	Cherry, black	Water (with lemon)
Apple cider	Cucumber	Vegetable juice
Apricot	Grapefruit	(corresponding
Carrot	Orange	with highlighted
Celery	Prune	vegetables)

Avoid

Tomato

Spices

Type Bs do best with warming herbs, such as ginger, horseradish, curry, and cayenne pepper. The exceptions are white and black pepper, which contain problem lectins. On the reverse side, sweet herbs tend to be stomach irritants, so avoid barley malt sweeteners, corn syrup, cornstarch, and cinnamon. The exceptions are white and brown sugar, honey, and molasses, which respond in a neutral way to the Type B digestive system. You may eat these sugars in moderation. You also may eat small quantities of chocolate, but consider it a condiment, not a main course!

Highly Beneficial

CAYENNE	GINGER
PEPPER	HORSERADISH
CURRY	PARSLEY

Neutral

Agar	Brown rice syrup	Chives
Anise	Capers	Chocolate
Arrowroot	Caraway	Clove
Basil	Cardamom	Coriander
Bay leaf	Carob	Cream of tartar
Bergamot	Chervil	Cumin

Dill
Dulse
Garlic
Honey
Kelp
Maple syrup
Marjoram
Mint
Miso
Molasses
Mustard (dry)
Nutmeg
Oregano
Paprika

Pepper,
    peppercorn
Pepper, red
    flakes
Peppermint
Pimiento
Rice syrup
Rosemary
Saffron
Sage
Salt
Savory
Soy sauce
Spearmint

Sugar, brown
Sugar, white
Tamarind
Tarragon
Thyme
Vanilla
Vinegar, apple cider
Vinegar, balsamic
Vinegar, red wine
Vinegar, white
Wintergreen

Avoid

Allspice
Almond extract
Barley malt
Cinnamon
Cornstarch
Corn syrup

Gelatin, plain
Pepper, black
    ground
Pepper, white
Tapioca

Condiments

Condiments are basically either neutral or bad for all types. Type Bs can handle just about every common condiment except ketchup (with its dangerous tomato lectins), but common nutritional sense would suggest that you limit your intake of foods that provide no real benefit.

Neutral

Apple butter
Jam (from acceptable fruits)
Jelly (from acceptable fruits)

Mayonnaise
Mustard
Pickles, dill

Pickles, kosher
Pickles, sour
Pickles, sweet
Relish

Salad dressing (low-fat, from
acceptable ingredients)
Worcestershire sauce

Avoid

Ketchup

Herbal Teas

Type Bs don't reap overwhelming benefits from most herbal teas, and only a few are harmful. Overall, Type Bs play things to a draw. They stay in balance with commonsense teas—ginger to warm, peppermint to soothe the digestive tract, and so on.

Ginseng is highly recommended for Type Bs because it seems to have a positive effect on the nervous system. Be aware, though, that it can act like a stimulant, so drink it early in the day.

Licorice is particularly good for Type Bs. It has antiviral properties that work to reduce your susceptibility to autoimmune diseases. Also, many Type Bs experience a drop in blood sugar after meals (hypoglycemia), and licorice helps regulate blood sugar levels.

More recently, I've discovered that licorice is a fairly powerful elixir for people suffering from chronic fatigue syndrome (see chapter 9).

Highly Beneficial

GINGER
GINSENG
LICORICE
LICORICE ROOT*
PARSLEY

PEPPERMINT
RASPBERRY LEAF
ROSE HIPS
SAGE

Do not use without your doctors permission.

Neutral

Alfalfa	Elder	Strawberry leaf
Burdock	Green tea	Thyme
Catnip	Hawthorn	Valerian
Cayenne	Horehound	Vervain
Chamomile	Mulberry	White birch
Chickweed	Saint-John's-wort	White oak bark
Dandelion	Sarsaparilla	Yarrow
Dong quai	Slippery Elm	Yellow dock
Echinacea	Spearmint	

Avoid

Aloe	Hops	Senna
Coltsfoot	Linden	Shepherd's purse
Corn silk	Mullein	Skullcap
Fenugreek	Red clover	
Gentian	Rhubarb	
Goldenseal		

Miscellaneous Beverages

Type Bs do best when they limit their beverages to herbal and green teas, water, and juice. Although beverages like coffee, regular tea, and wine do no real harm, the goal of the Blood Type Diet is to maximize your performance, not to keep it in neutral. If you're a caffeinated coffee or tea drinker, try replacing these beverages with green tea, which has caffeine but also provides some antioxidant benefits.

Highly Beneficial

TEA, GREEN

Neutral

Beer	Tea, black regular
Coffee, decaf	Wine, red
Coffee, regular	Wine, white
Tea, black decaf	

Avoid

Liquor, distilled	Soda, cola	Soda, other
Seltzer water	Soda, diet	

Meal Planning for Type B

An asterisk (*) denotes that the recipe follows.

THE FOLLOWING sample menus and recipes will give you an idea of a typical diet beneficial to Type Bs. They were developed by Dina Khader, M.S., R.D., a nutritionist who has used the Blood Type Diets successfully with her patients.

These menus are moderate in calories and balanced for metabolic efficiency in Type Bs. The average person will be able to maintain weight comfortably and even lose weight by following these suggestions. However, alternative food choices are provided if you prefer lighter fare or wish to limit your caloric intake and still eat a balanced, satisfying diet. (The alternative food is listed directly across from the food it replaces.)

Occasionally you will see an ingredient in a recipe that appears on your avoid list. If it is a very small ingredient (such as a dash of spice), you may be able to tolerate it, depending on your condition and whether you are strictly adhering to the diet. However, the meal selections and recipes are generally designed to work very well for Type Bs.

As you become more familiar with the Type B Diet recommendations, you'll be able to easily create your own menu plans and adjust favorite recipes to make them Type B–friendly.

STANDARD MENU ▪	WEIGHT-CONTROL ALTERNATIVES ▪

SAMPLE MEAL PLAN 1

Breakfast

Membrane Fluidizer Cocktail (optional)	
2 slices Ezekiel bread	1 slice Ezekiel bread
with	
*Yogurt-Herb Cheese	
poached egg	
green tea	

Lunch

Greek salad: lettuce, cucumber,
    scallions, celery, feta cheese,
    oil, and lemon
banana
iced herbal tea

Midafternoon snack

*Quinoa Applesauce Cake	scoop low-fat cottage
herbal tea	cheese with pear
	slices

Dinner

*Lamb/Asparagus Stew	broiled lamb chop
*Saffron Brown Rice	asparagus
steamed vegetables (broccoli, Chinese cabbage, etc.)	
frozen yogurt	
(wine if desired)	

S A M P L E   M E A L   P L A N   2

Breakfast
Membrane Fluidizer Cocktail
  (optional)
rice bran cereal with banana
  and skim milk
grape juice
coffee

Lunch
thin slice of cheese (Swiss or   2 slices turkey breast
  Munster), thin slice of turkey   1 slice spelt bread
  breast   mustard only
2 slices spelt bread
mustard or mayonnaise
green salad
herbal tea

Midafternoon snack
fruit-juice-sweetened yogurt
herbal tea

Dinner
*Broiled Fish
steamed vegetables
*Roasted Yams with Rosemary
mixed fresh fruit
herbal tea or coffee
(red or white wine if desired)

S AMPLE MEAL PLAN 3

Breakfast
Membrane Fluidizer Cocktail
    (optional)
*Maple-Walnut Granola with   puffed rice with goat's
    goat's milk   milk
1 soft-boiled egg
grapefruit juice
green tea

Lunch
*Spinach Salad
½ cup water-packed tuna with   ½ cup plain tuna
    mayonnaise   1 slice Essene bread
2 rice cakes
herbal tea

Midafternoon snack
*Apricot Fruit Bread   low-fat yogurt with
apple   raisins
coffee or tea

Dinner
*Scrumptious Fettuccine Alfredo
green salad
frozen yogurt
herbal tea
(red or white wine if desired)

Recipes

YOGURT-HERB CHEESE

2 32-oz. containers of plain, nonfat yogurt
2 cloves minced garlic
1 teaspoon thyme
1 teaspoon basil
1 teaspoon oregano
Salt and pepper to taste
1 tablespoon olive oil

Spoon yogurt into an old pillowcase or cheesecloth. Tie the cheesecloth with string and allow the yogurt to drip over the kitchen sink or the bathtub for 4½ to 5 hours.
Remove yogurt from cheesecloth and mix it with all the spices and oil in a bowl. Cover and chill for 1 to 2 hours before serving. Great served with raw vegetables.

QUINOA APPLESAUCE CAKE

1¾ cup quinoa flour
1 cup currants or other (allowed) dried fruit
½ cup chopped pecans
½ teaspoon baking soda
½ teaspoon aluminum-free baking powder
½ teaspoon salt
½ teaspoon ground cloves
2 cups unsweetened, organic applesauce
1 large organic egg
1 cup Sucanat sugar or maple sugar
½ cup unsalted, sweet butter

Preheat oven to 350 degrees F. Sprinkle ¼ cup of the flour over the currants and nuts and set aside. Blend the baking soda, powder, salt, and cloves with the remaining quinoa flour.

Add the dried fruit and nut mix and the applesauce. Beat in the egg and mix the sugar and butter in thoroughly.

Spoon into an oiled 8 x 8–inch cake pan and bake for 40 to 45 minutes or until the cake tester inserted in the center comes out clean.

LAMB-ASPARAGUS STEW

1 pound fresh asparagus spears
½ pound free-range lamb meat, cubed
1 medium onion, chopped
3 tablespoons organic, sweet unsalted butter
1 cup water
salt, pepper to taste
juice of 1 lemon

Cut asparagus spears in 2-inch lengths, discarding tough portion at bottom. Wash and drain.

Sauté meat and onions in butter until light brown. Add water, salt and spices. Cook until tender. Add asparagus. Simmer for 15 minutes or until tender. Add lemon juice.

Makes 2 servings.

SAFFRON BROWN RICE

3 tablespoons extra-virgin olive oil
1 large Spanish onion or red onion
1 teaspoon ground coriander
1 teaspoon nutmeg
2 cardamom pods (use seeds from inside only)

1 teaspoon saffron threads
2 tablespoons rose water (found in Middle Eastern stores)
2 cups brown basmati rice
4 cups filtered water (boiling)

Heat the oil and sauté onion with all spices except saffron for 10
minutes on low heat. In a separate dish crush the saffron threads
and add to simmering mixture.

Add half the rose water to the onion mixture. Simmer for another
15 minutes and then add the rice with boiling water. Cook for
35 to 40 minutes. Just before serving add the rest of the rose
water.

Makes 4 servings.

BROILED FISH
*RECIPE BY CHERYL MILLER

6 tablespoons unsalted butter, ghee, or oil
1 teaspoon hot pepper sauce
1 tablespoon fresh brown garlic
4 slices of your favorite fillet
1 cup of puffed rice cereal, crushed
2 tablespoons fresh parsley chopped

Melt butter, add hot pepper sauce and brown garlic. Pour 4 teaspoons into a glass rectangular baking dish. Arrange fillets,
sprinkle with crumbs. Add rest of the butter mixture on top of
fillets.

Broil 10 to 15 minutes. Sprinkle with parsley. Serve immediately.

Makes 4 servings.

**My patient and friend Cheryl Miller is a wonderful cook. She supplied
this recipe, and it's just delicious.*

ROASTED YAMS WITH ROSEMARY

5 to 6 medium yams, quartered
¼ cup extra-virgin olive oil
1 tablespoon fresh rosemary or 2 teaspoons dried
Dash cayenne or Cajun spice

Blend everything together and put into a Pyrex dish. Bake in the
oven at 350 to 375 degrees F for 1 hour. This is a wonderful
dish to have with a green salad or roasted vegetables.
Makes 4 servings.

MAPLE-WALNUT GRANOLA

4 cups rolled oats
1 cup rice bran
½ cup dried cranberries
½ cup dried currants
1 cup chopped walnuts
1 teaspoon vanilla extract
¼ cup organic canola oil
¾ cup maple syrup

Preheat oven to 250 degrees F. In a large mixing bowl combine
the oats, rice bran, dried fruit, nuts, and vanilla. Add the oil
and stir evenly.
Pour in maple syrup and mix well until evenly moistened. Mixture should be crumbly and sticky. Spread mixture in a cookie
tray and bake for 90 minutes, stirring every 15 minutes for
even toasting until the mixture is golden brown and dry.
Cool well and store in airtight container.

SPINACH SALAD

2 bunches fresh spinach
dash of salt to taste
1 bunch scallions, chopped
juice of 1 lemon
¼ tablespoon olive oil
pepper to taste

Wash spinach well. Drain and chop. Sprinkle with salt. After a few minutes, squeeze excess water. Add green onions, lemon juice, oil, salt, and pepper. Serve immediately.
Makes 6 servings.

APRICOT FRUIT BREAD

1¼ cup plain nonfat yogurt
1 organic egg
½ cup apricot conserves (fruit juice sweetened)
2 cups brown rice flour
1 teaspoon ground nutmeg
1¼ teaspoon baking soda
1 cup chopped, dried, unsulfured apricots
(or any other dried fruit)
½ cup currants

Lightly grease a standard-size loaf pan with butter and preheat oven to 350 degrees F. In a medium-size bowl, combine the yogurt, egg, and jam. Add 1 cup of flour and half of the spices plus soda. Stir until batter is evenly moist. Add remaining flour and spices. If consistency feels too thick you can add a few drops of cold water to the mixture. Fold in apricots and currants. Pour batter into greased loaf pan and bake for 40 to 45 minutes until done.
Remove bread from the pan and cool on a wire rack.
Makes approximately 8 servings.

SCRUMPTIOUS FETTUCCINE ALFREDO

8 ounces rice or spelt fettuccine/linguine
1 tablespoon extra-virgin olive oil
¾ cup buttermilk
⅓ cup plus 2 tablespoons Parmesan cheese (grated)
¼ cup sliced scallions
2 tablespoons chopped, fresh basil or 1 teaspoon dried
¼ teaspoon garlic powder or freshly pressed garlic
¼ teaspoon finely shredded lemon peel

Cook pasta according to package directions to the al dente stage. Drain; immediately return to pan. Add olive oil; toss to coat the pasta.

In same pan as pasta, add buttermilk, ⅓ cup Parmesan cheese, scallions, basil and garlic. Cook everything together over medium-high heat until bubbly, stirring constantly.

Decorate with 2 tablespoons Parmesan cheese and fresh basil. Serve with lemon.

Makes 4 side dishes.

Type B
Supplement Advisory

THE ROLE OF SUPPLEMENTS—be they vitamins, minerals, or herbs—is to add the nutrients that are lacking in your diet, and to provide extra protection where you need it. The supplement focus for Type Bs is:

- Fine-tuning an already balanced diet
- Improving insulin efficiency
- Strengthening viral immunity
- Improving brain clarity and focus

Type Bs are a special (you might say lucky) case. For the most part, you can avoid major diseases by following your Blood Type Diet. Because your diet is so rich in vitamin A, vitamin B, vitamin E, vitamin C, calcium, and iron, there is no need for supplementation of these vitamins and minerals. So enjoy your unique status—but follow your diet!

The following are the few supplements that can benefit Type Bs.

Beneficial

MAGNESIUM

While the other blood types risk calcium deficiency, Type Bs risk magnesium deficiency. Magnesium is the catalyst for the metabolic machinery in Type Bs. It's the match head—what makes Type Bs metabolize carbohydrates more efficiently. Since you are so efficient in assimilating calcium, you risk creating an imbalance between your levels of calcium and magnesium. Should this occur, you find yourself more at risk for viruses (or otherwise lowered immunity), fatigue, depression, and, potentially, nervous disorders. In these instances, perhaps a trial of magnesium supplementation (300–500 mg) should be considered. Also, many Type B children are plagued with eczema, and magnesium supplementation can often be beneficial.

Any form of magnesium is fine, although more patients report a laxative effect with magnesium citrate than with the other forms. An excessive amount of magnesium could, at least theoretically, upset your body's calcium levels, so be sure that you consume high-calcium foods as well, such as cultured dairy products. The key is balance!

Best Magnesium-Rich Foods for Type Bs

all recommended green vegetables,
grains, and legumes

Herbs/Phytochemicals
Recommended for Type Bs

L I C O R I C E *(Glycyrrhiza glabra).* Licorice is a plant widely used by herbalists around the world. It contains at least four benefits— as a treatment for stomach ulcers, as an antiviral agent against the herpes virus, to treat chronic fatigue syndrome, and to combat hypoglycemia.

Licorice is a plant to be respected: large doses in the wrong person can cause sodium retention and elevated blood pressure. If you are Type B and suffer from hypoglycemia, a condition where the blood sugar drops after a meal, drink a cup or two of licorice tea after meals. If you suffer from chronic fatigue syndrome, I recommend that you use licorice preparations, other than DGL and licorice tea, only under the guidance of a physician. Licorice freely used in its supplemental form can be toxic.

D I G E S T I V E   E N Z Y M E S . If you are a Type B who is not used to eating meat or dairy foods, you may experience some initial difficulties adapting to your diet. Take a digestive enzyme with your main meals for a while, and you'll adjust more readily to concentrated proteins. Bromelain, an enzyme found in pineapples, is available in supplemental form at many health food stores, usually in the 4x strength.

A D A P T O G E N I C   H E R B S . Adaptogenic herbs increase concentration and memory retention, sometimes a problem for Type Bs with nervous or viral disorders. The best are Siberian ginseng *(Eleutherococcus senticosus)* and *Ginkgo biloba,* both widely available in pharmacies and health food stores. Siberian ginseng has been shown in Russian studies to increase the speed and accuracy of teletype operators. *Ginkgo biloba* is currently the most frequently prescribed drug of any kind in Germany, where more than 5 million people take it daily.

Ginkgo increases the microcirculation to the brain, which is why it is often prescribed to the elderly. It is currently being promoted as a brain stimulant, a pick-me-up for the mind.

LECITHIN. Lecithin, a blood enhancer found principally in soy, allows the cell-surface B antigens to move around more easily and better protect the immune system. Type Bs should seek this benefit from lecithin granules, not soy itself, as soy doesn't have the concentrated effect. Using the Membrane Fluidizer Cocktail that I mentioned in the Type B Diet is a good habit to develop, as it allows you to get an excellent stimulant for your immune system in a rather pleasant way.

Type B Stress/Exercise Profile

THE TYPE B response to stress represents a balance of the nervous mental activity of Type A and the more physically aggressive reactions of Type O. Type Bs temper each of these qualities and so respond with harmony and balance—harnessing the best qualities of the other blood types.

The Type B response to stress is an evolutionary sophistication demanded by a multidimensional environment. Human beings needed the physical endurance required to conquer new lands, as well as the skills and patience to develop those lands. Remember, early Type Bs were represented by both nomads and agrarians.

As a Type B, you confront stress very well for the most part, because you blend more easily into unfamiliar situations. You're less confrontational than Type Os, but more physically charged than Type As.

Type Bs do well with exercises that are neither too aerobically intense nor completely aimed at mental relaxation. The ideal balance for many Type Bs consists of moderate activities that involve other people—such as group hiking, biking excursions, the less aggressive martial arts, tennis, and aerobics classes. You don't do as well when the sport is fiercely competitive—such as squash, football, or basketball.

The most effective exercise schedule for Type B should be three days a week of more intense physical activity and two days a week of relaxation exercises.

EXERCISE	DURATION	FREQUENCY
AEROBICS	45–60 min.	3x week
TENNIS	45–60 min.	3x week
MARTIAL ARTS	30–60 min.	3x week
CALISTHENICS	30–45 min.	3x week
HIKING	30–60 min.	3x week
CYCLING	45–60 min.	3x week
SWIMMING	30–45 min.	3x week
BRISK WALKING	30–60 min.	3x week
JOGGING	30–45 min.	3x week
WEIGHT TRAINING	30–45 min.	3x week
GOLF	60 min.	2x week
TAI CHI	45 min.	2x week
HATHA YOGA	45 min.	2x week

Type B
Exercise Guidelines

FOR PHYSICAL EXERCISE

The three components of a high-intensity exercise program are the warm-up period, the aerobic exercise period, and a cool-down period. A warm-up is very important to prevent injuries, because it brings blood to the muscles, readying them for exercise, whether it is walking, running, biking, swimming, or playing a sport. A warm-up should include stretching and flexibility movements to prevent muscle and tendon tears.

The exercise can be divided into two basic types: isometric

exercises, in which stress is created against stationary muscles; and isotonic exercises, such as calisthenics, running, or swimming, which produce muscular resistance through a range of movement. Isometric exercises can be used to tone up specific muscles, which can then be further strengthened by active isotonic exercise. Isometrics may be performed by pushing or pulling an immovable object or by contracting or tightening opposing muscles.

To achieve maximum cardiovascular benefits from aerobic exercise, you must elevate your heartbeat to approximately 70 percent of your maximum heart rate. Once that elevated rate is achieved during exercise, continue exercising to maintain that rate for thirty minutes. This regimen should be repeated at least three times each week.

To calculate your maximum heart rate:

1. Subtract your age from 220.
2. Multiply the difference by 70 percent (.70). If you are over sixty years of age, or in poor physical condition, multiply the remainder by 60 percent (.60).
3. Multiply the remainder by 50 percent (.50). For example, a healthy fifty-year-old woman would subtract 50 from 220, for a maximum heart rate of 170. Multiplying 170 by .70 would give her 119 beats per minute, which is the top level she should strive for. Multiplying 170 by .50 would give her the lowest number in her range.

FOR RELAXATION EXERCISES
Tai chi and yoga are the perfect way to balance the more physical activities of your week.

Tai chi chuan, or tai chi, is an exercise that enhances the flexibility of body movement. The slow, graceful, elegant gestures of tai chi chuan routines hardly resemble the original hand and foot blows, blocks, and parries they represent. In China, tai chi is practiced daily by groups who gather in public squares to perform the movements in unison. Tai chi can be a very effective relaxation technique, although it takes concentration and patience to master.

Yoga combines inner rectitude with breath control and postures designed to allow for complete concentration without distraction by worldly concerns. Hatha yoga is the most common form of yoga practiced in the West.

If you learn basic yoga postures, you can create a routine best suited to your lifestyle. However, some patients have told me that they are concerned that adopting yoga practices may conflict with their religious beliefs. They fear that the practice of yoga implies that they have adopted Eastern mysticism. I respond, "If you eat Italian food, does that make you Italian?" Meditation and yoga are what you make of them. Visualize and meditate on those subjects that are relevant to you. The postures are neutral; they are just timeless and proven movements.

Simple Yoga Relaxation Techniques

Yoga begins and ends with relaxation. We contract our muscles constantly, but rarely do we think of doing the opposite—letting go and relaxing. We can feel better and be healthier if we regularly release the tensions left behind within the muscles by the stresses and strains of life.

The best position for relaxation is lying on your back. Arrange your arms and legs so that you are completely comfortable in your hips, shoulders, and back. The goal of deep relaxation is to let your body and mind settle down to soothing calmness, in the same way that an agitated pool of water eventually calms to stillness.

Begin with abdominal breathing. As a baby breathes, its abdomen moves, not its chest. However, many of us grow to unconsciously adopt the unnatural and inefficient habit of restrained chest breathing. One of the aims of yoga is to make you aware of the true center of breathing. Observe the pattern of your breathing. Is your breathing fast, shallow, and irregular, or do you tend to hold your breath? Allow your breathing to revert to a more natural pattern—full, deep, regular, and with no constriction. Try to isolate just your lower breathing muscles; see if you can breathe without moving your chest. Breathing exercises are always done smoothly and without any strain. Place one hand on your navel and feel the movement of your breathing. Relax your shoulders.

Start the exercise by breathing out completely. When you inhale, pretend that a heavy weight, such as a large book, is resting on your navel, and that by your inhalation, you are trying to raise this imaginary weight up toward the ceiling.

Then, when you exhale, simply let this imaginary weight press down against your abdomen, helping you to exhale. Exhale more air out than you normally would, as if to "squeeze" more air out of your lungs. This will act as a yoga stretch for the diaphragm and further help to release tension in this muscle. Bring your abdominal muscles into play here to assist. When you inhale, direct your breath down so deeply that you are lifting an imaginary heavy weight back upward toward the ceiling. Try to completely coordinate and isolate the abdominal breath with no chest or rib movement.

A Final Note:
The Personality Question

EARLY TYPE Bs, confronted with new lands, unfamiliar climates, and the intermingling of races, had to be flexible and creative in order to survive. Type Bs required less ordered and harmonious conformity than the settled Type As, as well as less of the hunter's purposefulness that characterized Type Os.

These same characteristics exist in the very cells of Type Bs. Biologically, Type Bs are more flexible than Type Os, Type As, or Type ABs—less vulnerable to many diseases common to the others. The Type B who lives in harmony, working, exercising and eating in a balanced way, is the essence of a survivor.

In many ways, Type Bs have the best of all possible worlds. They have elements of the mental, more sensitively agitated activity of the Type A, with the sheer physical reactions and aggression of the Type O. Perhaps Type Bs relate more easily to different personality types because they are by genetic nature more in harmony and thus feel less inclined to challenge and confront. They can see others' points of view; they are empathetic.

A notable statistic: while Type B blood constitutes only 9 percent of the United States population, some 30 to 40 percent of all self-made millionaires are Type B!

The Chinese, Japanese, and many other Asian societies are composed of a high number of Type Bs. Chinese medicine—ancient, natural, and complex—places a great emphasis on balancing the physiological and emotional states. Unbridled joy (a desirable state for most Westerners) is viewed by Chinese physicians as being dangerous to the balance of the heart. Balance and harmony; this is a very Type B kind of medicine.

Traditional Jewish populations are primarily Type B, regardless of their geographic locations. Jewish religion and culture represent the blending of mind, soul, and matter. In Jewish tradition, intelligence, peace, and spirituality live side by side with a forceful physicality and readiness for battle. To many people, this seems like a contradiction. It is really the harmonious energies of the Type B in action.

SEVEN

Blood Type

AB

Plan

TYPE AB: *The Enigma*

- MODERN MERGING OF A AND B
- CHAMELEON'S RESPONSE TO CHANGING ENVIRONMENTAL AND DIETARY CONDITIONS
- SENSITIVE DIGESTIVE TRACT
- OVERLY TOLERANT IMMUNE SYSTEM
- RESPONDS BEST TO STRESS SPIRITUALLY, WITH PHYSICAL VERVE AND CREATIVE ENERGY
- AN EVOLUTIONARY MYSTERY

The Type AB Diet

BLOOD TYPE AB is less than a thousand years old, rare (2 to 5 percent of the population), and biologically complex. It doesn't fit comfortably into any of the other categories. Multiple antigens make Type ABs sometimes A-like, sometimes B-like, and sometimes a fusion of both—kind of a blood type centaur.

This multiplicity of qualities can be positive or negative, depending on the circumstances, so the Type AB Diet requires that you read your foods lists very carefully, and familiarize yourself with both the Type A and Type B diets to better understand the parameters of your own diet.

Essentially, most foods which are contraindicated for either Type A or Type B are probably bad for Type AB—although there are some exceptions. Panhemaglutinans, which are lectins capable of agglutinating all of the blood types, seem to be better tolerated by Type ABs, perhaps because the lectins' reaction is diminished by the double A and B antibodies. Tomatoes are an excellent example. Type A and Type B cannot tolerate the lectins, while Type AB eats tomatoes with no discernible effect.

Type ABs are often stronger and more active than the more sedentary Type As. This extra dollop of élan vital may be because their genetic memories still contain fairly recent remnants of their steppe-dwelling Type B ancestors.

The Weight-Loss Factor

WHEN IT COMES to gaining weight, Type ABs reflect the mixed inheritance of their A and B genes. Sometimes that means special problems. For example, you have Type A's low stomach acid, along with Type B's adaptation to meats. So, although you are genetically programmed for the consumption of meats, you lack enough stomach acid to metabolize them efficiently, and the meat you eat tends to get stored as fat. For weight loss, you should restrict your consumption of meats, eating small amounts that you can supplement with vegetables and tofu.

Your Type B propensities cause the same insulin reaction when you eat kidney or lima beans, corn, buckwheat, or sesame seeds (although your Type A side makes you friendly to lentils and peanuts). Inhibited insulin production causes hypoglycemia, a lowering of blood sugar after meals, and leads to less efficient metabolism of foods.

Type ABs lack the severe reaction of Type Os and Type Bs to wheat gluten. But again, for weight-loss purposes, you should avoid wheat, which tends to make your muscle tissue more acidic. Type ABs utilize calories most efficiently when your tissue is somewhat alkaline.

FOODS THAT ENCOURAGE WEIGHT GAIN

RED MEAT	*poorly digested*
	stored as fat
	toxifies intestinal tract
KIDNEY BEANS	*inhibit insulin efficiency*
	cause hypoglycemia
	slow metabolic rate
LIMA BEANS	*inhibit insulin efficiency*
	cause hypoglycemia
	slow metabolic rate
SEEDS	*cause hypoglycemia*
CORN	*inhibits insulin efficiency*
BUCKWHEAT	*causes hypoglycemia*
WHEAT	*decreases metabolism*
	inefficient use of calories
	inhibits insulin efficiency

FOODS THAT ENCOURAGE WEIGHT LOSS

TOFU	*promotes metabolic efficiency*
SEAFOOD	*promotes metabolic efficiency*
DAIRY	*improves insulin production*
GREEN VEGETABLES	*improve metabolic efficiency*

KELP	*improves insulin production*
PINEAPPLE	*aids digestion*
	stimulates intestinal mobility

USE THESE GUIDELINES ALONG WITH YOUR ENTIRE TYPE AB DIET RECOMMENDATIONS.

Meats and Poultry

BLOOD TYPE AB		WEEKLY ▪ IF YOUR ANCESTRY IS		
Food	*Portion**	*African*	*Caucasian*	*Asian*
LEAN RED MEATS	4–6 OZ. *(men)* 2–5 OZ. *(women and children)*	1–3X	1–3X	1–3X
POULTRY	4–6 OZ. *(men)* 2–5 OZ. *(women and children)*	0–2X	0–2X	0–2X

The portion recommendations are merely guidelines that can help refine your diet according to ancestral propensities.

When it comes to eating meat and poultry, Type ABs borrow characteristics from both Type A and Type B. Like Type A, you do not produce enough stomach acid to effectively digest too much animal protein. Yet the key for you is portion size and frequency. Type ABs need some meat protein, especially the kinds of meat that represent your B-like heritage—lamb, mutton, rabbit, and turkey, instead of beef. The lectin that irritates the blood and digestive tracts of Type Bs has the same effect on you, so stay away from chicken.

Also avoid all smoked or cured meats. These foods can cause stomach cancer in people with low levels of stomach acid, the trait you share with Type As.

Highly Beneficial

LAMB	RABBIT
MUTTON	TURKEY

Neutral

Liver
Pheasant

Avoid

Bacon	Cornish Hens	Partridge
Beef	Duck	Pork
Beef, ground	Goose	Veal
Buffalo	Ham	Venison
Chicken	Heart	Quail

Seafood

BLOOD TYPE AB	WEEKLY ▪ IF YOUR ANCESTRY IS			
Food	*Portion*	*African*	*Caucasian*	*Asian*
ALL RECOMMENDED SEAFOOD	4–6 oz.	3–5x	3–5x	4–6x

There are a wide variety of seafoods for Type ABs, and it is an excellent source of protein for you. Like Type A, you have trouble digesting the lectins found in sole and flounder. You also share the Type A susceptibility to breast cancer. If you have a family history of breast cancer, introduce snails into your diet. The edible snail, *Helix pomatia,* contains a powerful lectin that specifically agglutinates mutated A-like cells for two of the most common forms of breast cancer (see chapter 10). This is a positive kind of agglutination; the snail lectin gets rid of sick cells.

Highly Beneficial

ALBACORE	OCEAN PERCH	SARDINE
(TUNA)	PICKEREL	SEA TROUT
COD	PIKE	SHAD
GROUPER	PORGY	SNAIL
HAKE	RAINBOW	STURGEON
MACKEREL	TROUT	
MAHIMAHI	RED SNAPPER	
MONKFISH	SAILFISH	

Neutral

Abalone	Salmon	Swordfish
Bluefish	Scallop	Tilefish
Carp	Shark	Weakfish
Catfish	Silver Perch	Whitefish
Caviar	Smelt	White perch
Herring (fresh)	Snapper	Yellow Perch
Mussels	Squid (calamari)	

Avoid

Anchovy	Flounder	Octopus
Barracuda	Frog	Oysters
Beluga	Haddock	Sea Bass
Bluegill Bass	Halibut	Shrimp
Clam	Herring (pickled)	Sole
Conch	Lobster	Striped Bass
Crab	Lox (smoked	Turtle
Crayfish	salmon)	Yellowtail
Eel		

Dairy and Eggs

BLOOD TYPE AB		WEEKLY ▪ IF YOUR ANCESTRY IS		
Food	*Portion*	*African*	*Caucasian*	*Asian*
EGGS	1 EGG	3–5X	3–4X	2–3X
CHEESES	2 OZ.	2–3X	3–4X	3–4X
YOGURT	4–6 OZ.	2–3X	3–4X	1–3X
MILK	4–6 OZ.	1–6X	3–6X	2–5X

For dairy foods, Type ABs can put on the "B" hat. You benefit from dairy foods, especially cultured and soured products—yogurt, kefir, and non-fat sour cream—which are more easily digested.

The primary factor you have to watch out for is excessive mucus production. Like Type As, you already produce a lot of mucus, and you don't need more. Watch for signs of respiratory problems, sinus attacks, or ear infections, which might indicate you should cut back on the dairy foods.

Eggs are a very good source of protein for Type ABs. Although they're very high in cholesterol, and Type ABs (like Type As) have some susceptibility to heart conditions, research has shown that the biggest culprits are not cholesterol-containing foods but rather saturated fats.

However, when you eat eggs, you can increase your protein and lower your cholesterol intake by using two egg whites for every one egg yolk. (Note that the lectin found in the chicken muscle is not present in eggs.)

Highly Beneficial

COTTAGE CHEESE	GOAT CHEESE	RICOTTA
FARMER	GOAT MILK	SOUR CREAM
FETA	KEFIR	(NON-FAT)
	MOZZARELLA	YOGURT

Neutral

Casein	Gouda	Skim or 2% milk
Cheddar	Gruyère	Soy cheese*
Colby	Jarlsburg	Soy milk*
Cream cheese	Monterey jack	String cheese
Edam	Munster	Swiss
Emmenthal	Neufchatel	Whey

Good dairy alternatives

Avoid

American cheese	Buttermilk	Provolone
Blue cheese	Camembert	Sherbet
Brie	Ice cream	Whole milk
Butter	Parmesan	

Oils and Fats

BLOOD TYPE AB		WEEKLY ∎ IF YOUR ANCESTRY IS		
Food	Portion	African	Caucasian	Asian
OILS	1 TABLESPOON	1–5X	4–8X	3–7X

Type ABs should use olive oil rather than animal fats, hydrogenated vegetable fats, or other vegetable oils. Olive oil is a monounsaturated fat that is believed to contribute to lower blood cholesterol. You may also use small amounts of ghee, a semifluid clarified butter popular in India, in your cooking.

Highly Beneficial

OLIVE OIL

Neutral

Canola oil   Linseed (flaxseed) oil
Cod liver oil   Peanut oil

Avoid

Corn oil   Sesame oil
Cottonseed oil   Sunflower oil
Safflower oil

Nuts and Seeds

BLOOD TYPE AB		WEEKLY • IF YOUR ANCESTRY IS		
Food	*Portion*	*African*	*Caucasian*	*Asian*
NUTS AND SEEDS	6–8 NUTS	2–5X	2–5X	2–3X
NUT BUTTERS	I TABLESPOON	3–7X	3–7X	2–4X

Nuts and seeds present a mixed picture for Type ABs. Eat them in small amounts and with caution. Although they can be a good supplementary protein source, all seeds contain the insulin-inhibiting lectins that make them a problem for Type Bs. On the other hand, you share the Type A preference for peanuts, which are powerful immune boosters.

Type ABs also tend to suffer from gallbladder problems, so nut butters are preferable to whole nuts.

Highly Beneficial

NUTS, CHESTNUTS   PEANUT BUTTER
PEANUTS   WALNUTS

Neutral

Almond butter	Nuts, cashews	Nuts, macadamia
Nuts, almonds	Nuts, hickory	Nuts, pignola
Nuts, Brazil	Nuts, litchi	Nuts, pistachio

Avoid

Nuts, filberts	Sesame butter	Sunflower butter
Poppy seeds	(tahini)	Sunflower seeds
Pumpkin seeds	Sesame seeds	

Beans and Legumes

BLOOD TYPE AB		WEEKLY ▪ IF YOUR ANCESTRY IS		
Food	*Portion*	*African*	*Caucasian*	*Asian*
ALL BEANS AND LEGUMES	CUP, DRY	3–5X	2–3X	4–6X

Beans and legumes are another mixed bag for Type ABs. For example, lentil beans are an important cancer-fighting food for Type ABs, although they are not advised for Type Bs. In particular, lentils are known to contain cancer-fighting antioxidants. On the other hand, kidney and lima beans, which slow insulin production in Type As, have the same effect in Type ABs.

Highly Beneficial

BEANS, NAVY	BEANS, SOY
BEANS, PINTO	LENTILS, GREEN
BEANS, RED	

Neutral

Beans, broad	Beans, copper	Beans, green
Beans, cannellini	Beans, northern	Beans, jicama

Beans, snap	Beans, white	Peas, green
Beans, string	Lentils, domestic	Peas, pods
Beans, tamarind	Lentils, red	

Avoid

Beans, aduke	Beans, fava	Beans, lima
Beans, azuki	Beans, garbanzo	Peas, black-eyed
Beans, black	Beans, kidney	

Cereals

BLOOD TYPE AB		WEEKLY ▪ IF YOUR ANCESTRY IS		
Food	*Portion*	*African*	*Caucasian*	*Asian*
ALL CEREALS	I CUP, DRY	2–3X	2–3X	2–4X

Guidelines for Type ABs favor both Type A and Type B recommendations. Generally, you do well on grains, even wheat, but need to limit your wheat consumption because the inner kernel of the wheat grain is highly acid forming for Type ABs. Wheat is also not advised if you are trying to lose weight. Type ABs with a pronounced mucus condition caused by asthma or frequent infections should also limit wheat consumption, as wheat causes mucus production. You'll have to experiment for yourself to determine how much wheat you can eat. Here we're not talking about stomach acid, but the acid/alkaline balance in your muscle tissues. Type ABs do best when their tissues are slightly alkaline. While the inner kernel of wheat grain is alkaline in Type Os and Type Bs, it becomes acidic in Type As and Type ABs.

Limit your intake of wheat germ and bran to once a week. Oatmeal, soy flakes, millet, farina, ground rice and soy granules are good Type AB cereals, but you must avoid buckwheat and corn.

Highly Beneficial

MILLET	RICE BRAN	RYEBERRY
OAT BRAN	RICE, PUFFED	SPELT
OATMEAL		

Neutral

Amaranth	Farina	Soy flakes
Barley	Granola	Soy granules
Cream of rice	Grape nuts	Wheat bran
Cream of wheat	Seven-grain	Wheat germ
Familia	Shredded wheat	

Avoid

Buckwheat	Cornmeal	Kasha
Cornflakes	Kamut	

Breads and Muffins

BLOOD TYPE AB	DAILY ▪ IF YOUR ANCESTRY IS			
Food	Portion	African	Caucasian	Asian
BREADS, CRACKERS	I SLICE	0–IX	0–IX	0–IX
MUFFINS	I MUFFIN	0–IX	0–IX	0–IX

The Type AB guidelines for eating breads and muffins are similar to those for cereals and grains. They are generally favorable foods, but if you produce excessive mucus or are overweight, these conditions make whole wheat inadvisable. Soy and rice flour are good substitutes for you. Be aware that sprouted wheat breads sold commercially often contain small amounts of sprouted wheat and are basically whole wheat breads. Read the ingredient labels. Avoid corn muffins and corn bread. Although Essene and

Ezekiel breads (found in health food stores) are sprouted wheat breads, the gluten lectin is destroyed in the sprouting process.

Highly Beneficial

BROWN RICE BREAD	MILLET RICE CAKES	SOY FLOUR BREAD
ESSENE BREAD	100% RYE BREAD	SPROUTED WHEAT BREAD
EZEKIEL BREAD	RYE CRISPS	WASA BREAD
FIN CRISP	RYE VITA	

Neutral

Bagels, wheat	Ideal Flat Bread	Spelt bread
Durum wheat	Matzos, wheat	Wheat bran muffins
Gluten-free bread	Multi-grain bread	
High-protein bread	Oat bran muffins	Whole wheat bread
	Pumpernickel	

Avoid

Corn muffins

Grains and Pasta

BLOOD TYPE AB		WEEKLY ▪ IF YOUR ANCESTRY IS		
Food	*Portion*	*African*	*Caucasian*	*Asian*
GRAINS	I CUP, DRY	2–3X	3–4X	3–4X
PASTA	I CUP, DRY	2–3X	3–4X	3–4X

Type AB benefits from a diet rich in rice rather than pasta, although you may have semolina or spinach pasta once or twice a week. Again, avoid corn and buckwheat in favor of oats and rye. Limit your intake of bran and wheat germ to once a week.

Highly Beneficial

FLOUR, OAT	RICE, BASMATI
FLOUR, RICE	RICE, BROWN
FLOUR, RYE	RICE, WHITE
FLOUR, SPROUTED WHEAT	RICE, WILD

Neutral

Couscous	Flour, Graham	Pasta, semolina
Flour, bulgur wheat	Flour, spelt	Pasta, spinach
Flour, Durum wheat	Flour, white	Quinoa
Flour, gluten	Flour, whole wheat	

Avoid

Buckwheat kasha
Flour, barley
Pasta, artichoke
Soba noodles

Vegetables

BLOOD TYPE AB	DAILY ▪ ALL ANCESTRAL TYPES	
Food	*Portion*	
RAW VEGETABLES	1 CUP, PREPARED	3–5X
COOKED OR STEAMED	1 CUP, PREPARED	3–5X

Fresh vegetables are an important source of phytochemicals, the natural substances in foods that have a tonic effect in cancer and heart disease prevention—diseases that afflict Type As and Type ABs more often as a result of weaker immune systems. They should be eaten several times a day. Type ABs have a wide selection—nearly all the vegetables that are good for either Type A or Type B are good for you as well.

The one exception is the panhemaglutinan in tomatoes, which affects all blood types. Since Type ABs have so much blood type material and the lectin isn't specific, you seem able to avoid the ill effects. I've tested Type ABs who were eating a lot of tomatoes, and their Indican Scales were clear.

Type ABs should make tofu a regular part of their diet, in combination with small amounts of meat and dairy. Tofu also has well-acknowledged cancer-fighting benefits.

Like Type Bs, you must avoid fresh corn and all corn-based products.

Highly Beneficial

BEET LEAVES	EGGPLANT	POTATOES,
BEETS	GARLIC	SWEET
BROCCOLI	KALE	SPROUTS,
CAULIFLOWER	MUSHROOM,	ALFALFA
CELERY	MAITAKE	TEMPEH
COLLARD	MUSTARD	TOFU
GREENS	GREENS	YAMS, ALL
CUCUMBER	PARSLEY	TYPES
DANDELION	PARSNIPS	

Neutral

Arugula	Cabbage, red	Chicory
Asparagus	Cabbage, white	Coriander
Bamboo shoots	Caraway	Daikon
Bok choy	Carrots	Endive
Cabbage, Chinese	Chervil	Escarole

Fennel
Fiddlehead ferns
Ginger
Horseradish
Kohlrabi
Leek
Lettuce, Bibb
Lettuce, Boston
Lettuce, iceberg
Lettuce, mesclun
Lettuce, romaine
Mushroom,
    abalone
Mushroom,
    domestic
Mushroom,
    Portobello

Mushroom,
    shiitake
Mushroom, tree
Mushroom, oyster
Mushroom, Enoki
Okra
Olives, green
Olives, Greek
Olives, Spanish
Onions, green
Onions, red
Onions, Spanish
Onions, yellow
Potatoes, red
Potatoes, white
Pumpkin
Radicchio

Rappini
Rutabaga
Scallion
Seaweed
Shallots
Snow peas
Spinach
Sprouts, Brussels
Squash, all types
Swiss chard
Tomato
Turnips
Water chestnut
Watercress
Zucchini

Avoid

Artichoke,
    domestic
Artichoke,
    Jerusalem
Avocado
Corn, white

Corn, yellow
Lima beans
Olives, black
Peppers, green
Peppers, jalapeño
Peppers, red

Peppers, yellow
Radishes
Sprouts, mung
Sprouts, radish

Fruits

BLOOD TYPE AB	DAILY ▪ ALL ANCESTRAL TYPES	
Food	*Portion*	
ALL RECOMMENDED FRUITS	1 FRUIT OR 3–5 OZ.	3–4X

Type ABs inherit mostly Type A intolerances and preferences for certain fruits. Emphasize the more alkaline fruits, such as grapes, plums, and berries, which can help to balance the grains that are acid forming in your muscle tissues.

Type ABs don't do particularly well on certain tropical fruits—in particular mangoes and guava. But pineapple is an excellent digestive aid for Type ABs.

Oranges also should be avoided, even though they may well be among your favorites. Oranges are a stomach irritant for Type ABs, and they also interfere with the absorption of important minerals. Lest you get confused, let me reiterate that the acid/alkaline reaction happens two different ways—in the stomach and in the muscle tissues. When I say that acidic oranges are a stomach irritant for Type ABs, I'm talking about the stomach irritation they can cause in the sensitive, alkaline Type AB stomach. Although stomach acid is generally low in Type ABs, the acid contained in oranges irritates the delicate stomach lining. Grapefruit is closely related to oranges and is also an acidic fruit, but it has positive effects on the Type AB stomach, exhibiting alkaline tendencies after digestion. Lemons also are excellent for Type ABs, aiding digestion and clearing mucus from the system.

Since vitamin C is an important antioxidant, especially for stomach cancer prevention, eat other vitamin C–rich fruits, such as grapefruit or kiwi.

The banana lectin interferes with Type AB digestion. I recommend substituting other high-potassium fruits such as apricots, figs, and certain melons.

Highly Beneficial

CHERRIES	GRAPES,	LEMONS
CRANBERRIES	CONCORD	LOGANBERRIES
FIGS, DRIED	GRAPES, GREEN	PINEAPPLES
FIGS, FRESH	GRAPES, RED	PLUMS, DARK
GOOSEBERRIES	GRAPEFRUIT	PLUMS, GREEN
GRAPES, BLACK	KIWI	PLUMS, RED

Neutral

Apples	Melon, canang	Nectarines
Apricots	Melon,	Papayas
Blackberries	cantaloupe	Peaches
Blueberries	Melon, casaba	Pears
Boysenberries	Melon, Christmas	Plantains
Currants, black	Melon, Crenshaw	Prunes
Currants, red	Melon, honeydew	Raisins
Dates	Melon, musk	Raspberries
Elderberries	Melon, Spanish	Strawberries
Kumquat	Melon,	Tangerines
Limes	watermelon	

Avoid

Bananas	Oranges	Rhubarb
Coconuts	Persimmons	Starfruit
Guava	Pomegranates	(carambola)
Mangoes	Prickly pears	

Juices and Fluids

BLOOD TYPE AB	DAILY ▪ ALL ANCESTRAL TYPES	
Food	*Portion*	
ALL RECOMMENDED JUICES	8 oz.	2–3X
WATER	8 oz.	4–7X

Type AB should begin each day by drinking a glass of warm water with the freshly squeezed juice of half a lemon to cleanse the system of mucus accumulated while sleeping. The lemon water also aids elimination. Follow with a diluted glass of grapefruit or papaya juice.

Stress high-alkaline fruits juices such as black cherry, cranberry, or grape.

Highly Beneficial

CABBAGE	CRANBERRY
CARROT	GRAPE
CELERY	PAPAYA
CHERRY, BLACK	

Neutral

Apple	Pineapple
Apple cider	Prune
Apricot	Water (with lemon)
Cucumber	Vegetable juice (corresponding
Grapefruit	with highlighted vegetables)

Avoid

Orange

Spices

Sea salt and kelp should be used in place of salt. Their sodium content is low—a concern for Type AB—and kelp has immensely positive heart and immune system benefits. It also is useful for weight control. Miso, made from soy, is very good for type ABs, and makes a delicious soup or sauce.

Avoid all pepper and vinegar because they are acidic. Instead of vinegar, use lemon juice with oil and herbs to dress vegetables or salads.

And don't be afraid to use generous amounts of garlic. It's a potent tonic and natural antibiotic, especially for Type ABs.

Sugar and chocolate are allowed in small amounts. Use them as you would condiments.

Highly Beneficial

CURRY	MISO
GARLIC	PARSLEY
HORSERADISH	

Neutral

Agar	Dulse	Savory
Arrowroot	Honey	Soy sauce
Basil	Kelp	Spearmint
Bay leaf	Maple syrup	Sugar, brown
Bergamot	Marjoram	Sugar, white
Brown rice syrup	Mint	Tamari
Cardamom	Molasses	Tamarind
Carob	Mustard (dry)	Tarragon
Chervil	Nutmeg	Thyme
Chive	Paprika	Turmeric
Chocolate	Peppermint	Vanilla
Cinnamon	Pimiento	Vinegar, apple
Clove	Rice syrup	cider
Coriander	Rosemary	Vinegar, balsamic
Cream of tartar	Saffron	Vinegar, red wine
Cumin	Sage	Wintergreen
Dill	Salt	

Avoid

Allspice	Gelatin, plain	Pepper, red flakes
Almond extract	ground	Pepper, white
Anise	Pepper, black	Tapioca
Barley malt	Pepper, cayenne	Vinegar, white
Capers	Pepper,	
Cornstarch	peppercorn	
Corn syrup		

Condiments

Be sure to avoid all pickled condiments, due to a susceptibility to stomach cancer. Also avoid ketchup, which contains vinegar.

Neutral

Jam (from acceptable fruits)
Jelly (from acceptable fruits)
Mayonnaise
Mustard

Salad dressing (low-fat, from acceptable ingredients)

Avoid

Ketchup
Pickles, dill
Pickles, kosher
Pickles, sweet

Pickles, sour
Relish
Worcestershire sauce

Herbal Teas

Herbal tea should be employed by Type ABs to rev up the immune system and build protections against cardiovascular disease and cancer. Alfalfa, burdock, chamomile, and echinacea are immune-system boosters. Hawthorn and licorice root are highly recommended for cardiovascular health. Green tea has enormous positive effects on the immune system. Dandelion, burdock root, and strawberry leaf teas will aid your absorption of iron and prevent anemia.

Highly Beneficial

ALFALFA	GINGER	LICORICE ROOT*
BURDOCK	GINSENG	ROSE HIPS
CHAMOMILE	GREEN TEA	STRAWBERRY
ECHINACEA	HAWTHORN	LEAF

Do not use without your doctor's permission.

Neutral

Catnip	Mulberry	Spearmint
Cayenne	Parsley	Thyme
Chickweed	Peppermint	Valerian
Dandelion	Raspberry leaf	Vervain
Dong quai	Sage	White birch
Elder	Saint-John's-wort	White oak bark
Goldenseal	Sarsaparilla	Yarrow
Horehound	Slippery elm	Yellow dock

Avoid

Aloe	Hops	Senna
Coltsfoot	Linden	Shepherd's purse
Corn silk	Mullein	Skullcap
Fenugreek	Red clover	
Gentian	Rhubarb	

Miscellaneous Beverages

Red wine is good for Type ABs because of its positive cardiovascular effects. A glass of red wine every day is believed to lower the risk of heart disease for both men and women.

A cup or two a day of regular or decaffeinated coffee increases your stomach acid and also has the same enzymes found in soy. Alternate coffee and green tea for the best combination of benefits.

Highly Beneficial

COFFEE, REGULAR
COFFEE, DECAF
TEA, GREEN

Neutral

Beer	Wine, red
Seltzer water	Wine, white
Soda, club	

Avoid

Liquor, distilled	Soda, diet	Tea, black decaf
Soda, cola	Soda, other	Tea, black regular

Meal Planning for Type AB

Asterisk (*) indicates the recipe follows.

THE FOLLOWING SAMPLE menus and recipes will give you an idea of a typical diet beneficial to Type ABs. They were developed by Dina Khader, M.S., R.D., a nutritionist who has used the Blood Type Diets successfully with her patients.

These menus are moderate in calories and balanced for metabolic efficiency in Type ABs. The average person will be able to comfortably maintain weight and even lose weight by following these suggestions. However, alternative food choices are provided if you prefer lighter fare or wish to limit your caloric intake and still eat a balanced, satisfying diet. (The alternative food is listed directly across from the food it replaces.)

Occasionally you will see an ingredient in a recipe that appears on your avoid list. If it is a very small ingredient (such as a dash of spice), you may be able to tolerate it, depending on your condition and whether you are strictly adhering to the diet. However, the meal selections and recipes are generally designed to work very well for Type ABs.

As you become more familiar with the Type AB Diet recommendations, you'll be able to easily create your own menu plans and adjust favorite recipes to make them Type AB-friendly.

STANDARD MENU ■   **WEIGHT-CONTROL**
                              ALTERNATIVES ■

SAMPLE MEAL PLAN I

Breakfast
water with lemon (on rising)
8 ounces diluted grapefruit juice
2 slices Ezekiel bread   I slice Ezekiel bread
*Yogurt-Herb Cheese   I poached egg
coffee

Lunch
4 ounces sliced turkey breast
2 slices rye bread   I slice rye bread or
Caesar salad   2 rye crisps
2 plums
herbal tea

Midafternoon snack
*Tofu Cheesecake   ½ cup low-fat yogurt
iced herbal tea   with fruit

Dinner
*Tofu Omelet
stir-fried vegetables
mixed-fruit salad
decaffeinated coffee
(red wine if desired)

SAMPLE MEAL PLAN 2

Breakfast
water with lemon (on rising)
diluted grapefruit juice

*Maple-Walnut Granola with
   soy milk
coffee

Lunch
*Tabbouleh
bunch of grapes or apple
iced herbal tea

Midafternoon snack
*Carob Chip Cookies   honeydew melon with
coffee or herbal tea   scoop cottage cheese

Dinner
*Grilled Rabbit
*String Bean Salad
basmati rice   steamed broccoli and
frozen yogurt   cauliflower
decaffeinated coffee
(red wine if desired)

SAMPLE MEAL PLAN 3

Breakfast
water with lemon (on rising)
diluted grapefruit juice
1 poached egg
2 slices Essene bread with   1 slice Essene bread
   organic almond butter   with low-sugar jam
coffee

Lunch
*Tofu-Sardine Fritters
or   tofu-vegetable stir-fry
*Tofu-Pesto Lasagna

mixed-green salad
2 plums
herbal tea

Midafternoon snack
fruit-juice-sweetened yogurt

Dinner
broiled salmon with fresh dill
   and lemon
*Saffron Brown Rice   asparagus
*Spinach Salad
decaffeinated coffee
(red wine if desired)

Recipes

YOGURT-HERB CHEESE

2 32-ounce containers of plain, nonfat yogurt
2 cloves minced garlic
1 teaspoon thyme
1 teaspoon basil
1 teaspoon oregano
1 tablespoon olive oil

Spoon yogurt into an old pillowcase or cheesecloth. Tie the
   cheesecloth with string and allow the yogurt to drip over a
   kitchen sink or a bathtub for 4½ to 5 hours.
Remove yogurt from cheesecloth and mix it with all the spices
   and oil in a bowl. Cover and chill for 1 to 2 hours before serving. Great served with raw vegetables.

TOFU CHEESECAKE (BAKED)
(RECIPE BY YVONNE CHAPMAN)

1 ½ pounds pressed tofu
⅔ cup soy milk
¼ teaspoon salt (optional)
2 teaspoons fresh lemon juice
grated rind of one lemon
1 teaspoon vanilla extract

Blend all ingredients together.

PIE CRUST

¾ cup whole meal flour (or rye flour)
½ cup oatmeal
½ teaspoon salt
½ cup oil
2 tablespoons cold water

Combine ingredients, stir in oil, then water, until mixture holds together. Press over bottom and sides of an 8-inch pie pan. Prick bottom several times with a fork. Fill pie crust with tofu mixture and bake at 300 degrees F for 30 to 45 minutes. Makes approximately 8 servings.

TOFU OMELET

1 pound soft tofu, drained and mashed
5–6 Portobello mushrooms, sliced
½ pound grated scallions
1 teaspoon mirin or sherry for cooking
1 teaspoon wheat-free tamari soy sauce
1 tablespoon fresh parsley, chopped

1 teaspoon brown rice flour
4 organic eggs, lightly beaten
choice of allowable seasonings to taste
2 teaspoons organic extra-virgin olive oil

Combine all the ingredients except for oil. Heat the oil in a large
frying pan. Pour in half the mixture and cover the pan. Cook
over low heat for approximately 15 minutes until egg is
cooked. Remove from pan and Keep warm.
Repeat the process and use the remainder of the mixture.
Serves 3 to 4.

MAPLE-WALNUT GRANOLA

4 cups rolled oats
1 cup rice bran
½ cup dried currants
½ cup dried cranberries
1 cup minced walnuts or almonds
1 teaspoon vanilla extract
¼ cup organic canola oil
¾ cup maple syrup

Preheat oven to 250 degrees F. In a large mixing bowl combine
the oats, rice bran, dried fruit, nuts, and vanilla. Add the oil
and stir evenly.
Pour in maple syrup and mix well until evenly moistened. Mixture should be crumbly and sticky. Spread mixture in a cookie
tray and bake for 90 minutes, stirring every 15 minutes for
even toasting until the mixture is golden brown and dry.
Cool well and store in airtight container.

TABBOULEH

1 cup millet, cooked
1 bunch green onions, chopped
4 bunches parsley, chopped
1 bunch mint, chopped, or 2 tablespoons dried mint
1 large cucumber, peeled and chopped (optional)
⅓ cup olive oil
juice of 3 lemons
1 tablespoon salt

Place millet in a large bowl. Add all chopped vegetables and mix well. Add oil, lemon juice, and salt. Serve over fresh green lettuce. Eat with lettuce leaves, tender grape leaves, or with a fork. Makes a refreshing appetizer or a picnic salad.
Makes 4 servings.

CAROB CHIP COOKIES

⅓ cup organic canola oil
½ cup pure maple syrup
1 teaspoon vanilla extract
1 organic egg
1 teaspoon baking soda
1¾ cups oat or brown rice flour
½ cup carob chips (unsweetened)

Oil two baking sheets and preheat oven to 375 degrees F. In a medium-size mixing bowl, combine the oil, maple syrup and vanilla. Beat the egg and stir into the oil mixture. Gradually stir in soda and flour to form a stiff batter. Fold in carob chips and drop the batter onto the baking sheets by the teaspoon. Bake for 10 to 15 minutes until cookie is lightly browned. Remove from oven and cool.
Makes 3½ to 4 dozen.

GRILLED RABBIT

2 rabbits
1 cup apple cider vinegar
1 small onion, chopped
2 teaspoons salt
¼ cup water
1 cup rice flour or crushed wheat-free bread crumbs
¼ teaspoon pepper
dash of cinnamon
⅓ cup margarine

Clean dressed rabbits and cut into serving pieces. Marinate meat in vinegar, onion, and salted water for a few hours before cooking. Drain.

Combine flour, salt and spices in a plate. Dip pieces in melted margarine, then in flour or crushed bread crumb mixture until well coated.

Grill in oven at 375 degrees F for 30 to 40 minutes.

Makes 4 to 6 servings.

STRING BEAN SALAD

1 pound green string beans
juice of 1 lemon
3 tablespoons olive oil
2 cloves garlic, crushed
2 to 3 teaspoons salt

Wash tender, fresh, green string beans. Remove stems and strings. Cut into 2-inch pieces.

Cook until tender by boiling in plenty of water. Drain. When cool, place in a salad bowl. Dress to taste with lemon juice, olive oil, garlic, and salt.

Makes 4 servings.

TOFU SARDINE FRITTERS
(RECIPE BY YVONNE CHAPMAN)

1 can deboned sardines
2 1-inch slices of medium or firm tofu
¼ teaspoon horseradish powder
dash of cider vinegar
olive oil

Mash sardines with a fork until fluffy. Mash tofu into the sardines.
   Sprinkle in the horseradish powder. Add a dash of vinegar.
   Continue mixing ingredients until well blended.
Form into small patties. Heat a small amount of olive oil in
   a heavy skillet. Brown both sides of patties, or alternatively
   brown under a grill. This recipe goes well with a salad.
Serves 2.

TOFU-PESTO LASAGNA

1 pound soft tofu, mashed with 2 tablespoons olive oil
1 cup shredded mozzarella cheese (part skim)
or part-skim ricotta
1 organic egg (optional)
2 packages frozen, chopped spinach or fresh, cut-up spinach
1 cup water
1 teaspoon salt
1 teaspoon oregano
9 rice or spelt lasagna noodles, cooked
4 cups pesto sauce (you may use less)

Mix tofu and cheese with egg, spinach, water, and seasonings.
   Layer 1 cup sauce in 9 x 13 baking dish. Layer noodles, then
   cheese mixture, and then sauce. Repeat and end with noodles
   and sauce on top. Bake in oven at 350 degrees F for 30 to 45
   minutes or until done.

SAFFRON BROWN RICE

3 tablespoons extra-virgin olive oil
1 large Spanish onion or red onion
1 teaspoon ground coriander
1 teaspoon nutmeg
2 cardamom pods (use only seeds inside)
1 teaspoon saffron threads
2 tablespoons rose water (found in Middle Eastern stores)
2 cups brown basmati rice
4 cups filtered water (boiling)

Heat the oil and sauté onion with all spices for 10 minutes on low heat. In a separate dish beat the saffron and add to rose water in a small bowl.

To the onion mixture, add 1 tablespoon rose water. Simmer for another 15 minutes and then add the rice with boiling water. Cook for 35 to 40 minutes. Just before serving add the rest of the rose water.

Makes 4 servings.

SPINACH SALAD

2 packages, fresh spinach
1 bunch scallions, chopped
Juice of 1 lemon
¼ tablespoon olive oil or flaxseed oil
Salt and pepper to taste
Hot pepper (optional)

Wash spinach well. Drain and chop. Sprinkle with salt. After a few minutes, squeeze excess water. Add scallions, lemon juice, oil, salt and pepper. Serve immediately.

Makes 6 servings.

Type AB
Supplement Advisory

THE ROLE OF SUPPLEMENTS—be they vitamins, minerals, or herbs—is to add the nutrients that may be lacking in your diet, and to provide extra protection where you need it. The supplement focus for Type ABs is:

- Supercharging the immune system
- Supplying cancer-fighting antioxidants
- Strengthening the heart

Type ABs present a somewhat mixed picture when it comes to supplements. Although you share the vulnerable immune system and disease susceptibilities of Type As, your Type AB diet fortunately provides a rich variety of nutrients with which to fight back.

For example, Type ABs get plenty of vitamin A, vitamin B-12, niacin, and vitamin E in their diets, receiving a dietary protection against cancer and heart disease. I would suggest further supplementation only if, for some reason, a Type AB isn't adhering to the diet. Even iron, which is seriously lacking in the Type A vegetarian diet, is readily available in Type AB foods. There are, however, some supplements that can benefit Type ABs.

VITAMIN C

Type ABs, who have higher rates of stomach cancer because of low stomach acid, can benefit from taking additional supplements of vitamin C. For example, nitrite, a compound that results from the smoking and curing of meats, could be a particular problem with Type ABs, because its cancer-causing potential is greater in people with lower levels of stomach acid. As an antioxidant, vitamin C is known to block this reaction (although you should still avoid smoked and cured foods). However, don't take this to mean that you should take massive amounts. I have found that Type ABs do not do as well on high doses (1,000 mg and up) of vitamin C because it tends to upset their stomachs. Taken over the course of a day, two to four capsules of a 250 mg supplement, preferably derived from rose hips, should cause no digestive problems.

Best C-Rich Foods for Type ABs

berries	cherries
grapefruit	lemon
pineapple	broccoli

ZINC (WITH CAUTION)
I have found that a small amount of zinc supplementation (as little as 3 mg/day) often makes a big difference in protecting Type AB children against infections, especially ear infections. Zinc supplementation is a double-edged sword, however. While small, periodic doses enhance immunity, long-term, higher doses depress it and can interfere with the absorption of other minerals. Be careful with zinc! It's completely unregulated and is widely available as a supplement, but you really shouldn't use it without a physician's advice.

Best Zinc-Rich Foods for Type ABs

recommended meats (especially dark-meat turkey)
eggs
legumes

SELENIUM
Selenium may be of value to Type ABs, as it seems to act as a component of the body's own antioxidant defenses. However, cases of selenium toxicity have been reported in people who have taken excessive supplements. Check with your physician before taking this mineral.

Herbs/Phytochemicals
Recommended for Type ABs

HAWTHORN *(Crataegus oxyacantha).* With a tendency toward heart disease, Type ABs will want to be serious about protecting their cardiovascular system. Following the Type AB diet will substantially reduce the risk, but if you have family members with heart disease or hardening of the arteries, you may want to take your preventive program a step further. A phytochemical with exceptional preventive capacities is found in the hawthorn tree *(Crataegus oxyacantha).* Hawthorn has a number of impressive antioxidant effects. It increases the elasticity of the arteries and strengthens the heart while also lowering blood pressure and exerting a mild solventlike effect upon the plaques in the arteries. Officially approved for pharmaceutical use in Germany, the actions of hawthorn are virtually unknown elsewhere. Extracts and tinctures are readily available through naturopathic physicians, health food stores, and pharmacies. I cannot praise this herb too highly. Official German government monographs show the plant to be completely free of any side effects. If I had my way, extracts of hawthorn would be used to fortify breakfast cereals, just as vitamins are.

IMMUNE-ENHANCING HERBS. Because the immune systems of Type AB tend to be vulnerable to viruses and infections, gentle immune-enhancing herbs such as purple coneflower *(Echinacea purpurea)* can help ward off colds or flus and may help optimize the immune system's anti-cancer surveillance. Many people take echinacea in liquid or tablet form. It is widely available. The Chinese herb huang-ki *(Astragalus membranaceous)* is also taken as an immune tonic, but is not as easy to find. In both herbs the active ingredients are sugars that act as mitogens to stimulate white blood cell proliferation. The white blood cells, you will remember, defend the immune system.

CALMING HERBS. Type ABs will do well to use mild herbal relaxants such as chamomile and valerian root. These herbs are available as teas and should be taken frequently. Valerian has a bit of a pungent odor, which actually becomes pleasing once you get used to it.

QUERCETIN. Quercetin is a bioflavonoid found abundantly in vegetables, particularly yellow onions. Quercetin supplements are widely available in health food stores, usually in capsules of 100 to 500 mg. Quercetin is a very powerful antioxidant, many hundreds of times more powerful than vitamin E. Quercetin makes a powerful addition to your cancer-prevention strategies.

MILK THISTLE *(Silybum marianum)*. Like quercetin, milk thistle is an effective antioxidant with the additional special property of reaching very high concentrations in the liver and bile ducts. Type ABs tend to suffer from digestive disorders, particularly of the liver and gallbladder. If your family has any history of liver, pancreas, or gallbladder problems, add a milk thistle supplement (easily found in most health food stores) to your protocol. Cancer patients who are receiving chemotherapy should use a milk thistle supplement to protect their liver from damage.

BROMELAIN *(Pineapple enzymes)*. If you are Type AB and suffer from bloating or other signs of poor absorption, take a bromelain supplement. This enzyme has a moderate ability to break down dietary proteins, helping the Type AB digestive tracts better assimilate them.

Type AB Stress/Exercise Profile

THE ABILITY to reverse the negative effects of stress lives in your blood type. As we discussed in chapter 3, stress is not in itself a problem; it's how you respond to stress. Type ABs have inherited the exact stress pattern of Type As. In this way, you are not at all B-like.

Type ABs react to the first stage of stress—the alarm stage—intellectually. Adrenally charged bulbs flash in your brain, producing anxiety, irritability, and hyperactivity. As the stress signals throb in your immune system, you grow weaker. The heightened sensitivity of your nervous system gradually frays your delicate protective antibodies. You're too weary to fight the infections and bacteria that are waiting to jump in like muggers trailing an intoxicated prey.

If, however, you adopt quieting techniques, such as yoga or meditation, you can achieve great benefits by countering negative stresses with focus and relaxation. Type ABs do not respond well to continuous confrontation, and need to consider and practice the art of stillness as a calming charm.

If Type ABs remain in their naturally tense state, stress can produce heart disease and various forms of cancer. Exercises that provide calm and focus are the remedy that pull the Type AB from the grip of stress.

Tai chi chuan, the slow-motion, ritualistic pattern of Chinese boxing; and hatha yoga, the timeless Indian stretching system, are calming, centering experiences. Moderate isotonic exercises, such as hiking, swimming, and bicycling, are favored for Type ABs. When I advise calming exercises, it doesn't mean you can't break a sweat. The key is really your mental engagement in your physical activity.

For example, heavy competitive sports and exercises will only exhaust your nervous energy, make you tense all over again, and leave your immune system open to illness or disease.

The following exercises are recommended for Type ABs. Pay special attention to the length of the sessions. To achieve a consistent release of tension and revival of energy, you need to perform one or more of these exercises three or four times a week.

EXERCISE	DURATION	FREQUENCY
TAI CHI	30–45 min.	3–5x week
HATHA YOGA	30 min.	3–5x week
AIKIDO	60 min.	2–3x week

GOLF	60 min.	2–3x week
CYCLING	60 min.	2–3x week
BRISK WALKING	20–40 min.	2–3x week
SWIMMING	30 min.	3–4x week
DANCE	30–45 min.	2–3x week
AEROBICS (LOW-IMPACT)	30–45 min.	2–3x week
HIKING	45–60 min.	2–3x week
STRETCHING	15 min.	every time you exercise

Type AB
Exercise Guidelines

TAI CHI CHUAN, or tai chi, is an exercise that enhances the flexibility of body movement. The slow, graceful, elegant gestures of tai chi chuan routines seem to mask the full-speed hand and foot blows, blocks, and parries they represent. In China, tai chi is practiced daily by groups who gather in public squares to perform the movements in unison. Tai chi can be a very effective relaxation technique, although it takes concentration and patience to master.

Yoga is also good for the Type AB stress pattern. It combines inner rectitude with breath control and postures designed to allow for complete concentration without distraction by worldly concerns. Hatha yoga is the most common form of yoga practiced in the West.

If you learn basic yoga postures, you can create a routine best suited to your lifestyle. Many Type ABs who have adopted yoga relaxation tell me that they will not leave the house until they do their yoga.

However, some patients have told me that they are concerned that adopting yoga practices may conflict with their religious beliefs. They fear that the practice of yoga implies that they have adopted Eastern mysticism. I respond, "If you eat Italian food, does that make you Italian?" Meditation and yoga are what you make of them. Visualize and meditate on those subjects that are relevant to you. The postures are neutral; they are just timeless and proven movements.

SIMPLE YOGA RELAXATION TECHNIQUES

Yoga begins and ends with relaxation. We contract our muscles constantly, but rarely do we think of doing the opposite—letting go and relaxing. We can feel better and be healthier if we regularly release the tensions left behind within the muscles by the stresses and strains of life.

The best position for relaxation is lying on your back. Arrange your arms and legs so that you are completely comfortable in your hips, shoulders, and back. The goal of deep relaxation is to let your body and mind settle down to soothing calmness, in the same way that an agitated pool of water eventually calms to stillness.

Begin with abdominal breathing. As a baby breathes, its abdomen moves, not its chest. However, many of us grow to unconsciously adopt the unnatural and inefficient habit of restrained chest breathing. One of the aims of yoga is to make you aware of the true center of breathing. Observe the pattern of your breathing. Is your breathing fast, shallow, and irregular, or do you tend to hold your breath? Allow your breathing to revert to a more natural pattern—full, deep, regular, and with no constriction. Try to isolate just your lower breathing muscles; see if you can breathe without moving your chest. Breathing exercises are always done smoothly and without any strain. Place one hand on your navel and feel the movement of your breathing. Relax your shoulders.

Start the exercise by breathing out completely. When you inhale, pretend that a heavy weight, such as a large book, is resting on your navel, and that by your inhalation, you are trying to raise this imaginary weight up toward the ceiling. Then, when you exhale, simply let this imaginary weight press down against your abdomen, helping you to exhale. Exhale more air out than you normally would, as if to "squeeze" more air out of your lungs. This will act as a yoga stretch for the diaphragm and help to further release tension in this muscle. Bring your abdominal muscles into play here to assist. When you inhale, direct your breath down so deeply that you are lifting an imaginary heavy weight back upward toward the ceiling. Try to completely coordinate and isolate the abdominal breath with no chest or rib movement.

Even if you perform more aerobic exercises during the course of your week, try to integrate the relaxing, soothing routines that will help you best manage your Type AB stress patterns.

A Final Note:
The Personality Question

TYPE AB followers of blood type–personality analysis love to boast that Jesus Christ was Type AB. Their evidence comes from blood tests conducted on the Shroud of Turin. It's a provocative idea, although I have my doubts, since Jesus was supposed to have lived a good one thousand years before the emergence of Type AB.

But that's Type AB for you. They don't always sweat the details. Type AB is a merging of the edgy, sensitive Type A with the more balanced and centered Type B. The result is a spiritual, somewhat flaky nature that embraces all aspects of life without being particularly aware of the consequences. These characteristics are clearly evident in Type AB blood. The Type AB immune system is the best friend to nearly every virus and disease on the planet. If Type O has high-tech security gates on its immune system, Type AB doesn't even have a lock on its door.

Naturally, these qualities make Type ABs very appealing and popular. It's easy to like people who welcome you with open arms, don't hold grudges when you disappoint them, and always say the most diplomatic thing in every situation. Not surprisingly, many healers and spiritual teachers are Type AB.

The problem is, since Type ABs' immune systems are so indiscriminate, you begin to suspect that they have no loyalty to any one group. Benedict Arnold, our nation's most famous traitor, was said to be Type AB.

On the positive side, Type ABs are considered some of the most captivating and interesting of the blood types. But their natural charisma can often lead to heartache. John F. Kennedy and Marilyn Monroe were Type ABs, and though long gone, both remain prominent. There was a public connection to them so intense that it haunts the American psyche to this day. But for all their luster, their charisma exacted a heavy toll.

Your Blood Type Health

EIGHT

Medical
Strategies

*The Blood
Type Connection*

Y NOW YOU ARE AWARE OF THE STRONG LINK BE-
tween your blood type and your health. I hope you are also beginning to see that you can exert meaningful control, even when
you have a susceptibility to a certain condition. Your Blood Type
Plan is the cornerstone to a lifetime of health.

In the next three chapters, we will talk in more detail about
the specific medical issues that concern everyone, and how you
can use your blood type information to make the best choices for
your health. We begin with the drugs and treatments that are
commonplace in modern life.

Drugs have been used as medicine for thousands of years.
When a shaman or witch doctor brewed a potion, that potion had
not only medical authority, but spiritual power. Although the infusion was often malodorous and vile, it contained magic, and the
patient would gladly drink the bitter brew in hope of a cure.

Not that much has changed.

Today physicians overprescribe medications, and we overuse
them. It's a serious problem. Yet unlike other naturopaths who reject the entire modern pharmacopoeia, I believe we must take a

more reasoned and flexible point of view. Most medical preparations are designed to be effective on a broad range of the population, and should be used to treat the most severe and potentially dangerous conditions.

But let us also keep medication in perspective: All drugs are poisons. The good drugs that man has discovered over the centuries are selective poisons. Many others are broader, less selective poisons. An excellent example of the latter is the diffuse arsenal of drugs used by oncologists for chemotherapy. In the process of destroying cancerous cells, many of these drugs indiscriminately attack healthy cells as well. (It is not my intention to vilify oncologists. This is just the state of the art.)

The good news is that chemotherapy sometimes works. The bad news is that sometimes chemotherapy works, but the patient dies of complications related to the treatment. It's a terrible conundrum.

Modern science has presented the medical community with a bewildering array of medications, and all of them are being prescribed by well-meaning physicians worldwide. But have we been careful enough in our use of antibiotics and vaccines? How do you know which medications are best for you, for your family, for your children?

Again, blood type holds the answer.

Over-the-Counter Medications

THERE IS A wide range of over-the-counter (OTC) medications designed for every common ailment—from headaches to aching joints to congestion to indigestion. On the face of it, these seem to be inexpensive, convenient, and effective remedies.

As a naturopathic physician, I try to avoid prescribing OTC medications whenever I can. In most cases, there are natural alternatives that work just as well or better. In addition, there are dangers inherent in using many OTC preparations, including:

- Aspirin's blood-thinning properties can be trouble for Type Os, who already have thin blood. Furthermore, they can mask the symptoms of a serious infection or illness.
- Antihistamines can raise blood pressure—a particular danger for Types A and AB. They can also cause sleeplessness and exacerbate prostate problems.
- Habitual use of laxatives actually can cause constipation, disrupting the natural process of elimination. They also can be harmful for people with Crohn's disease—primarily a Type O problem.
- Cough, throat, and chest remedies often have side effects, including high blood pressure, drowsiness, and dizziness.

Before you take an OTC remedy to treat a headache, cramps, or any other malady, investigate the possible causes of your problem. Often, it relates to your diet or stress. For example, you might ask:

- Is my headache a result of stress?
- Is my stomach discomfort caused by eating foods that are indigestible for my blood type?
- Are my sinus problems the result of mucus caused by eating too many mucus-generating foods? Or by eating histamine-releasing foods (such as wheat for Type O)?
- Is my flu virus the result of immune-system weaknesses?
- Is my congestion or bronchitis caused by an overproduction of mucus in my respiratory passages?
- Is my toothache caused by an infection that requires immediate medical treatment?
- Is my overreliance on commercial laxatives interfering with natural elimination and causing diarrhea?

I urge you to seek medical attention if your symptoms are chronic or particularly severe. Pain, weakness, coughs, fever, congestion, and diarrhea all can be signs of deeper problems. You might cover them up with medications, but you won't be addressing the root cause.

For occasional aches, pains and irregularities, the following remedies are excellent natural replacements for OTC drugs. They're available in many forms from your local health food store or natural nutrition center—including teas, compresses, liquid tinctures, extracts, powders, and capsules.

To make your own herbal tea, boil water and steep the natural herbs for about five minutes.

Please note the key indicating special considerations for each blood type.

KEY

●   Type O avoid

■   Type A avoid

▼   Type B avoid

†   Type AB avoid

★   Special note for all blood types

HEADACHE

chamomile	valerian
damiana ●	white willow bark (*salix*)
feverfew	

SINUSITUS

fenugreek ▼ †	thyme

ARTHRITIS

alfalfa ●	epsom salt bath
boswella	rosemary tea soak
calcium	

EARACHE

garlic-mullein-olive oil ear drops

TOOTHACHE

crushed garlic gum
  massage

oil of cloves gum
  massage

INDIGESTION, HEARTBURN

bladderwrack

ginger

bromelain (from pineapple)

goldenseal

gentian ● †

peppermint

CRAMPS, GAS

chamomile tea

peppermint tea

fennel tea

probiotic supplement

ginger

  with bifidus factor

NAUSEA

cayenne ▨

licorice root tea

ginger

FLU

arabino galactan

goldenseal

echinacea

rose hip tea

garlic

FEVER

catnip ■

vervain

feverfew

white willow bark

COUGH

coltsfoot ● ▼

linden ▼

horehound

SORE THROAT

fenugreek tea gargle ▼   stone root

goldenseal root and sage tea gargle

CONGESTION

licorice tea   nettle

mullein ▼   vervain

CONSTIPATION

aloe vera juice ● ▼ †   psyllium

fiber ★★   slippery elm

larch tree bark (ARA-6) ★

DIARRHEA

blueberries   *L. acidophilus* (yogurt culture)

elderberries   raspberry leaf

MENSTRUAL CRAMPS

Jamaican dogwood

★   Currently under patent, substance of larch tree bark
     in a powdered form is available from my office under
     the name ARA-6. It has been tested to be an excel-
     lent natural immune system booster. Furthermore, a
     substance in larch tree bark, called butyrate, is a safe
     and effective natural source of fiber for all blood
     types. For more information and orders, see Appen-
     dix F.

★★ Natural fiber is available in many fruits, vegetables,
     and grains. Be sure to check your blood type food list
     before you choose a fiber source.

Vaccines: The Blood Type Sensitivities

VACCINATION is an emotionally charged issue in both the conventional and alternative medical communities. From the more orthodox viewpoint, vaccination represents the first line of defense in preventive medicine. Increasing emphasis is being placed on mandatory universal vaccination by the federal, state, and local levels of government. What are the consequences of such a strategy?

Vaccines have been of unquestioned benefit to mankind, saving hundreds of thousands of lives and preventing needless suffering. In the rare circumstances where there have been problems, the vaccines have sometimes reacted badly with a particularly hypersensitive individual. Our knowledge of the immune system does not yet reveal if vaccines have more profound resonances, possibly lowering some of our innate immunities to cancer. Yet many public health officials and medical scientists behave as though it is somehow unpatriotic to question whether every new vaccine must be injected into the collective national bloodstream.

Meanwhile, the public remains confused. Parents want to know which vaccines, if any, their children should be exposed to. The elderly, the hypersensitive, pregnant women, and others worry about the effects of vaccinations. It shouldn't surprise you that there is no single answer for everyone. Your reaction to vaccines has a lot to do with your blood type.

Type O Vaccine Sensitivities

With all vaccines, parents of Type O children should be alert to any sign of inflammation, such as fever or joint pain, since the Type O immune system is prone to these reactions.

Avoid the injectable form of polio vaccine for Type O children, and opt instead for the oral preparation. Since Type Os have hyperactive immune systems, they do best with a less potent form of the vaccine.

Recently vaccinated Type O children should be watched carefully for a couple of days to ensure that there are no complications. Don't give them acetaminophen, the most commonly prescribed over-the-counter medication for vaccination-related problems (found in Tylenol). In my experience, Type O children seem to react poorly to this drug. A natural remedy that will work for Type Os is available at most health food stores. It is an herb called feverfew, derived from the common chrysanthemum flower *(Chrysanthemum parthenium)*. In liquid tincture form, feverfew can be given to a child every few hours. Four to eight drops of the tincture in a glass of juice is sufficient to achieve a positive effect.

If you are a pregnant woman with Type O blood, the flu vaccine holds special dangers, especially if the father of your baby is a Type A or Type AB. The flu vaccine could boost the presence of anti-A antibodies in your system, which could attack and damage your fetus.

Type A and Type AB Vaccine Sensitivities

Type A and Type AB children respond well to vaccines. A full vaccination program—including the whooping cough vaccine—should produce few side effects.

In contrast to Type O, Type A and Type AB children should take the injectable form of the polio vaccine because their digestive mucus does not react well to the oral polio vaccine.

Type B Vaccine Sensitivities

Type B children sometimes have severe neurological reactions to vaccinations. Parents should be acutely aware of any signal indicating a complication, be it an alteration in your child's walking or crawling gait, or a personality change of some kind. If you intend to vaccinate your Type B child, it is imperative that you make sure he or she is first completely healthy—free of colds, flu, or ear infections. Like Type Os, Type B children should use the oral form of polio vaccine.

Why do Type Bs tend to react so badly to vaccines? Type Bs produce an enormous number of B antigens in their nervous system. I believe a cross-reaction occurs in the Type B immune system when a vaccine is introduced that causes the body to turn and attack its own tissues. It may be the vaccine itself that causes this cross-reaction. Or perhaps it's one of the chemicals used to enhance the vaccine's effectiveness. It might even be the culture medium used to grow the vaccine. We just don't know yet.

Pregnant Type B women should also avoid the flu vaccine, especially if the father of the child is of Type A or Type AB blood. The flu vaccine could increase your production of anti-A antibodies, which could interfere with the healthy development of the fetus.

The Pros and Cons of Antibiotic Therapy

IF YOUR PHYSICIAN or your child's pediatrician often prescribes antibiotics for simple colds and flu, I have one piece of advice: Find another doctor.

The constant misuse of antibiotics is a leading factor in our growing inability to eradicate disease. The overuse of such wonder drugs promotes the development of progressively more resistant pathogens, which require ever stronger antibiotics to treat. Far more powerful than any of the antibiotics currently being manufactured is the natural prescription of proper diet, proper rest, and stress reduction.

Typically, there is a lag between the time you develop an infection and the time your body's immune system responds. It's like dialing the 911 emergency number; you know they aren't going to be at your door the second they answer your call. Antibiotics may get to an infection faster, but they hang up the phone on your body's own 911 emergency number—the immune system. Antibiotics basically cut off immune response; your body's responsibility for fighting an infection has been taken over by medication.

We race to treat fever with antibiotics, yet fever is generally a good sign. It indicates that your body's metabolic rate has kicked into overdrive, burning out invaders by making the environment as inhospitable to infectious organisms as it possibly can.

In my own practice I have discovered that a majority of people can eliminate an infection without the use of an antibiotic. Did you know that antibiotics only reduce the level of infection? Your body's immune system is still required to finish the battle. When you allow your body to go to war on its own terms, without antibiotic intervention, it develops not only a memory of specific antibodies to the current infection and any similar to it, but also the ability to fight more effectively the next time it is challenged or attacked.

A number of people are allergic to various antibiotics, but as a rule they produce few serious medical conditions. Very often, however, continued and heavy use of antibiotics destroys not only the infection, but all of the good bacteria in the digestive tract. Many people experience diarrhea, and quite often women become subject to recurring and persistent yeast infections. Supplements of a friendly digestive bacteria, *L. acidophilus*, may be taken in either tablets or yogurt to restore the proper balance of bacteria in the digestive tract.

There are, of course, times when an appropriate antibiotic is needed and should be used. If you are given an antibiotic, take a supplement of bromelain to ensure that your antibiotic spreads rapidly and penetrates tissue more readily. Pineapples contain this enzyme, so you may drink pineapple juice or take bromelain tablets when you're on a course of antibiotics.

Parents of sick children on antibiotics should set the alarm clock for three or four A.M. to administer an extra dose during the child's sleep cycle. This ensures a more rapid concentration of the drug to fight the infection.

Once more: If you need antibiotics, take them. If an infection becomes protracted, you certainly should consider using an antibiotic. I just think the body's immune system should be allowed to do what it's been created for—to resist.

Type O Antibiotic Sensitivities

Type Os should avoid penicillin-class antibiotics. The Type O immune system is more allergically sensitive to this class of drugs.

Also avoid sulfa-class drugs such as Bactrim. They can cause skin rashes in Type Os.

Try to avoid macrolide-class antibiotics. Erythromycin and the newer macrolides Biaxin and Zithromax can aggravate bleeding tendencies in Type Os. Be especially wary of this problem if you are currently taking blood-thinning medications such as Coumadin or Warferin.

Type A Antibiotic Sensitivities

Carbacephem-class antibiotics such as Lorabid seem to work well for Type As. There are very few side effects. Most Type As respond well to penicillin-class and sulfa-class antibiotics. These are preferable to tetracycline or the newer macrolide-class antibiotics.

If a macrolide-class antibiotic is prescribed for a Type A, Erythromycin is preferred over Zithromax or Clarythromycin. Both of these antibiotics can cause digestive problems and interfere with iron metabolism in the Type A system.

Type AB and Type B Antibiotic Sensitivities

Avoid quinolone-class antibiotics such as Floxin and Cipro if you can. If you must use them, take them (as Europeans do) in smaller doses than prescribed. Be aware of any sign of a nervous system disorder when taking a course of antibiotics, such as blurred vision, confusion, dizziness, or insomnia. Type AB and Type B should immediately discontinue the use of such medication and contact their physicians.

Antibiotic Therapy at the Dentist

It is standard practice for dentists to use antibiotics as a preventive measure against infection. Patients with mitral valve prolapse, a heart condition, are always given a course of antibiotics to guard against any possibility of bacterial infection and subsequent valve damage.

However, a recent study in the British medical journal *Lancet* found no benefit to a course of antibiotics for the majority of patients prior to invasive dental procedures. However, if you are a non-secretor (see Appendix E), you are at much greater risk than a secretor for infections following dental surgery. There are many more instances of streptococcal bacteria causing endocarditis (an inflammation of the lining of the heart muscle) and rheumatic fever in non-secretors, because they produce much lower levels of protective antibodies in the mucous membranes of the mouth and throat. Secretors, on the other hand, have higher levels of these IgA antibodies, which trap bacteria and destroy them before they can gain access to the bloodstream.

Non-secretors should always undertake preventive antibiotic therapy prior to any invasive dental procedure—from deep cleaning to oral surgery.

If you are Type O you may wish to opt out of antibiotic therapy, unless there is deep-rooted infection or the promise of heavy bleeding. Instead, try herbal medications with anti-strep activity, such as goldenseal *(Hydrastis canadensis).*

Type A, Type B, and Type AB may wish to discuss alternative therapies with their dentist or physician if they respond poorly to antibiotics.

Many dentists will refuse to treat a patient who declines the prophylactic use of antibiotics. If you are a healthy individual with no prior history of infections, you might want to consider going elsewhere for your dental work.

Surgery: Better Recovery

ANY INVASIVE PROCEDURE is a shock to your system. Never take it lightly, even if it is a minor surgery. Tune up your immune system in advance, no matter what your blood type.

Vitamins A and C have a profound effect on wound healing and minimize the formation of scar tissue. Every blood type can benefit from supplementation before surgery. Start taking vitamins A and C at least four or five days prior to surgery, and continue for at least a week afterward. All of my patients who have followed this recommendation report that both they and their surgeons were astonished at the rapidity of their recovery.

RECOMMENDED SURGICAL SUPPLEMENTATION PROTOCOL

Blood Type	Daily Vitamin C	Daily Vitamin A
TYPE O	2000 MG	30,000 IU
TYPE A	500 MG	10,000 IU
TYPE AB, TYPE B	1000 MG	20,000 IU

Type O Surgical Cautions

Type Os often experience greater blood loss than other blood types during and after surgery because they have lower levels of serum clotting factors. Make sure that you have plenty of vitamin K in your system before surgery; it is essential to clot formation. Kale, spinach, and collard greens contain ample amounts of this vitamin, although you might want to supplement your diet with liquid chlorophyll. Chlorophyll supplements are available at any health food store.

Type Os with a history of phlebitis or who are on a course of blood thinners should consult with their physicians as to any supplementation recommendations. (It's worth noting that the thinner blood of Type Os does not necessarily protect against blood clots. Phlebitis often starts as an inflammatory condition of the veins that affects blood flow.)

Type Os can also boost their immune systems and metabolism with strong physical activity. If it is realistic for you to pursue this prior to surgery, exercise will allow your body to deal with the stress of surgery much more effectively and heal more rapidly.

Type B Surgical Cautions

Type Bs are fortunate in that they are less likely to experience post-surgical complications. The vitamin protocol should be followed as already indicated.

Type Bs who are suffering from a weakened condition may also want to use immune-boosting herbal teas prior to surgery. Burdock root *(Arctium lappa)* and purple coneflower *(Echinacea purpurea)* are excellent immune boosters. A few cups of tea taken every day over a number of weeks can be a positive stimulant for your immune system.

Type A and Type AB Surgical Cautions

Type A and Type AB are both more prone to postsurgical bacterial infections. These infections can become a major stumbling block to recovery and can exacerbate an already difficult situation. I strongly suggest that Type A and Type AB adopt a blood-building, immune system–enhancing protocol of additional vitamin supplementation a week or two prior to surgery. Vitamin B-12, folic acid, and supplemental iron should all be taken daily along with the already suggested levels of vitamins A and C. The concentration of vitamins you need to achieve is difficult to squeeze out of the Type A and Type AB diets, so supplementation is best.

Floradix is a liquid iron and herb source that is both gentle on the digestive tract and highly assimilable. I highly recommend its use for iron supplementation since iron is usually an irritant to the digestive tracts of Type As and Type ABs. Floradix is found in most health food stores.

Avail yourselves of the two excellent immune-enhancing herbal teas, burdock root and echinacea. Drink a few cups daily of these herbal teas at least a couple of weeks prior to surgery.

More than the other blood types, Type As and Type ABs often experience profound physical, mental, and emotional stress because of the trauma of surgery. Relaxation techniques, such as meditation and visualization, can be of tremendous benefit to the more highly strung Type A and Type AB patient. By practicing these techniques, you can have a profound influence upon your own healing process. Some anesthesiologists will work with patients on visualizations while the patient is under anesthesia. I urge you to ask your doctor about this. It's a perfect method for Type As.

After the Surgery
Calendula succus (marigold) is used to help the wound heal and keep it clean. A solution of this homeopathic herb—a form of the marigold flower—is a wonderful healer for all cuts and scrapes in general. The juice has mild antibiotic properties and can be left on after application. Be sure you buy the juice, or *succus*, and not the *calendula* tincture, which has a high alcohol content. The tincture will really sting if you try to clean a wound with it.

As your incision heals and the stitches or staples are removed, a topical vitamin E preparation will minimize scar tissue formation and skin tightening. Many people just snip open a vitamin E capsule and smear it on, but oral supplements aren't formulated for use as skin healers. Use a topical cream or lotion blended for just this purpose.

Listen to Your Blood Type

THERE ARE MANY vitamins and herbal supplements that aid the body in both defending and healing itself. The recommended surgical supplementation is just the minimum you should do to protect and strengthen yourself.

Each of the Blood Type Diets contains pertinent information that allows you to make reasoned choices about what you should and should not allow yourself to eat and drink. All of these choices can have a profound effect on your health and the quality of your life.

By making knowledgeable choices about what is best for your body, you will be able to dramatically affect the course of both your treatment and recovery from surgery. This not only grants you greater control over your present circumstances, but enables you to ensure your future health.

Parents whose children are of vaccination age . . . people who have viral infections . . . those facing surgery—everyone can achieve benefits from an awareness of the blood type connection. It makes sense. It also solves the puzzle of why some people do very well with conventional treatments, while others suffer complications and pain. I urge you to put yourself in the position of being someone who does well.

Blood Type:

A Power

Over Disease

*E*VERYONE WHO GETS SICK WANTS TO KNOW "WHY ME?"
Even with our enormous technological arsenal, we often have no
certain answer to that question.

It has become clear, however, that there are individuals who
are more prone to certain diseases because of their blood type.
Perhaps this is the missing link—the way we can understand the
cellular causes of disease, and devise ways to combat and eliminate it more effectively.

Why Some People Are
Susceptible . . . and Some Are Not

CAN YOU REMEMBER being young and having a close friend who
wanted you to do something that you were reluctant to do? Take
a puff of a forbidden cigarette? Sneak a drink of whiskey from
your father's liquor cabinet? Did you take that puff? Drink that
whiskey?

If you did, you exhibited your susceptibility—your lack of resistance—to the suggestion of a friend.

Susceptibility, or lack of resistance, is the basic issue with most disease. Many microbes have the ability to mimic antigens that are considered friendly by the security force of a particular blood type. These clever mimics bypass the security guards and gain entry. Once in the system, they quickly overwhelm it and take control.

Don't you ever wonder why one person stays perfectly healthy while everyone else is falling prey to the latest cold or flu? It is because the healthy person's blood type is not susceptible to those particular invaders.

The Blood Type Connection

THERE ARE MANY causal factors for disease that are clearly influenced by blood type. For instance, Type As with a family history of cardiovascular disease should examine their diets very carefully. Red meats and saturated fats of all kinds are poor choices for a digestive tract ill suited to their processing, which results in higher levels of both triglycerides and cholesterol in Type As. The friendly Type A immune system is also more prone to cancer, since it has a hard time recognizing foes.

Type Os, as I've said, are very sensitive to the agglutinating lectin found in whole wheat. This lectin interacts with the lining of the Type O intestinal tract and produces additional inflammation. If you're Type O and suffer from Crohn's disease, colitis, or irritable bowel syndrome, wheat acts like a poison in your system. Although the Type O immune system is generally hardy, it is also limited. Original Type Os had fewer microbes to conquer, and the blood type does not adapt easily to the complex viruses prevalent today.

The disease profiles of Type Bs are independent of Type O and Type A by virtue of the idiosyncratic B antigens. They tend to be susceptible to slow-moving, sometimes bizarre viral diseases that don't manifest themselves for many years—such as multiple sclerosis and rare neurological ailments—sometimes triggered by the lectins in foods such as chicken and corn.

Type ABs have the most complex disease profile, since they possess both A-like and B-like antigens. Most of their disease susceptibilities are A-like, so if you had to categorize them you would say they were more A than B.

The blood type connection between good health and disease is a potent tool in our search for the best way to treat the body as it is meant to be treated.

Still, I must add a caveat, lest you think that I am proposing a magic formula. There are many factors in every individual life that contribute to disease. It would be overly simplistic and certainly foolish to suggest that blood type is the sole determining factor. If a Type O, a Type A, a Type B, and a Type AB each drank a cup of arsenic, each of them would die. By the same token, if four people of different blood types were all heavy smokers, they would all be susceptible to lung cancer.

The blood type information is not a panacea, but a meaningful refinement that will enable you to function at your peak.

Let's turn to the most common and troubling diseases and conditions for which we can identify a blood type relationship. Some blood type–disease relationships are more clearly defined than others. We are still learning. But every day blood type is revealed as a dominating factor—the previously missing link in our quest for health.

CATEGORIES*

- AGING DISEASES
- ALLERGIES
- ASTHMA AND HAY FEVER
- AUTOIMMUNE DISORDERS

Note: Cancer is such a complex topic that I have devoted an entire chapter to it, following this one.

- BLOOD DISORDERS
- CARDIOVASCULAR DISEASE
- CHILDHOOD ILLNESSES
- DIABETES
- DIGESTIVE ILLNESSES
- INFECTIONS
- LIVER DISEASE
- SKIN DISORDERS
- WOMEN/REPRODUCTION

Aging Diseases

ALL PEOPLE AGE, no matter what their blood type. But why do we age—and can we slow down the process? These questions have fascinated us for as long as we can remember. The promise of a Fountain of Youth has appeared in every century. Today, with our sophisticated medical technology and our increased knowledge of the factors that contribute to aging, we are closer to an answer.

But there's another question: Why do individual aging patterns differ so greatly? Why does the fifty-year-old runner, lean and seemingly fit, drop dead of a heart attack, while the eighty-nine-year old woman who has never broken a sweat in her life, remains hale and hardy? Why do some people develop Alzheimer's disease or dementia, while others do not? At what age does physical deterioration become inevitable?

We understand some pieces of the puzzle. Genetics play a role; unique variations in chromosomes contribute to susceptibilities that cause deterioration more rapidly in one person than in another. But these studies are incomplete.

I have discovered, however, a critical link between blood type and aging—specifically, a correlation between the agglutinating action of lectins and the two biggest physiological associations with aging—kidney failure and brain deterioration.

As we age we experience a gradual drop in kidney function so that by the time the average person reaches age seventy-two, his or her kidneys are operating at only 25 percent of their capacity.

Your kidney function is a reflection of the volume of blood that gets cleaned and recirculated into your bloodstream. This filtering system is very delicate—large enough for the various fluid elements of blood to go though, but small enough to prevent whole cells from passing through.

Consider the way the agglutinating actions of lectins gum up the works. Because the kidneys play a central role in the filtration of blood, the actions of many lectins can, over time, upset the delicate process. Those lectins that find their way into the bloodstream end up agglutinating and lodging in the kidneys. The process is similar to having a clogged drain. Over time, the filtration system ceases to function. As more and more agglutination occurs, less and less blood is able to be cleaned. It is a slow process, but ultimately deadly. Kidney failure is one of the leading causes of physical deterioration in the elderly.

The second large physiological association with aging occurs in the brain. Here lectins play an equally destructive role. Scientists have observed that the difference between an old brain and a young brain is that in an old brain many elements of neurons get tangled up. This tangling, which leads to dementia and overall deterioration (and might even be a factor in Alzheimer's disease) occurs very gradually over the decades of adult life.

How do lectins reach the brain? Remember, lectins come in all shapes and sizes; some are small enough to pass the blood-brain barrier. Once they reach the brain they begin to agglutinate the blood cells, gradually interfering with neuron activity. The process occurs over many decades, but eventually the neurons get tangled enough to have an effect on brain function.

It is clear to me that by reducing or eliminating the most harmful lectins from your diet, you can maintain healthier kidneys and brain function for a longer period of time. That is why some very old people remain mentally sharp and physically active.

A third way that lectins contribute to aging is their effects on our hormonal functions. It is well documented that as people age they have more trouble absorbing and metabolizing nutrients. That's one reason why elderly people often become malnourished, even when they are eating their normal diets. Dietary guidelines normally call for added supplementation for the elderly. But if agglutinating lectins are not overwhelming the system and interfering with hormonal activity, it is likely that elderly people can absorb nutrients as effectively as when they were younger.

I am not proposing that the Blood Type Solution is the Fountain of Youth! It is not a formula for reversing the effects of aging that have already occurred. But you can reduce cellular damage by reducing your lectin intake at any age. Most of all, your Blood Type Plan is designed to be age sparing—enabling you to slow down the process of aging during your entire adult life.

Allergies

Food Allergies

In my opinion, no area of alternative medicine is as shot full of humbug as the concept of food allergy. Complex and expensive tests are conducted on practically every patient, resulting in a list of foods to which that person is "allergic."

My own patients habitually term any reaction to something they've eaten a "food allergy," although most of the time it is not an allergy they are describing, but rather a food intolerance. If you have a problem with lactose in milk, for example, you are not allergic to it; you lack an enzyme to break it down. You are lactose intolerant, not lactose allergic. This intolerance does not necessarily mean you'll get sick if you drink milk. Type Bs who are lactose intolerant, for example, are often able to introduce milk products into their diets gradually. There are also products that add the lactose enzyme to milk products, making them more palatable for the intolerant.

A food allergy is a very different type of reaction that occurs, not in the digestive tract, but in the immune system. Your immune system literally creates an antibody to a food. The reaction is swift and harsh—rashes, swelling, cramps, or other specific symptoms that indicate your body is struggling to rid itself of the poisonous food.

Not everything in nature is perfectly cut and dried. Occasionally I'll come across a person who is allergic to a food that is on his Blood Type Diet. The solution: simply remove the offending food. The main point is that you have more to fear from the hidden lectins entering your system than you do from food allergies. You may not feel sick when you eat the food, but it is affecting your system nonetheless. Type As should also be aware that if they produce excessive mucus, it may appear to be an allergy when they should actually be avoiding mucus-producing foods.

Asthma and Hay Fever

TYPE OS WIN the allergy sweepstakes hands down! They are more likely to be asthma sufferers, and even hay fever, the bane of so many, appears to be specific to Type O blood. A wide range of pollens contain lectins that stimulate the release of the powerful histamines, and *boom!* Itching, sneezing, runny nose, wheezing, coughing, red, watery eyes—all allergy symptoms.

Many food lectins, especially wheat, interact with IgE (immunoglobin-E) antibodies found in the blood. These antibodies stimulate white blood cells called basophiles to release not only histamines, but other powerful chemical allergens called kinins. These can cause severe allergic reactions, swelling the tissues of the throat and constricting the lungs.

Asthma and hay fever sufferers really do best when they follow the diet recommended for their blood type. For example, Type Os who eliminate wheat often relieve many of their symptomatic behaviors, such as sneezing, respiratory problems, snoring, or persistent digestive disorders.

Type As have a different problem. Instead of environmental reactions, they often develop stress-related asthma as a result of their intense stress profiles (see the Type A Plan). When Type As suffer from excessive production of mucus caused by poor dietary choices, it makes the stress-related asthma worse. Type As, as you will remember, naturally produce copious amounts of mucus, and when they eat foods that are mucus producing (such as dairy), they suffer from too much mucus, which can exacerbate respiratory problems. In this case, when Type As are careful to avoid mucus-producing foods, and when the causes of the stress are addressed positively, their asthmatic condition always improves or is eliminated.

By design, Type Bs are not prone to developing allergies. They have a high allergy threshold, unless they eat the wrong foods. For example, the B-poisoning chicken and corn lectins will trigger allergies in even the most resistant Type Bs.

Type ABs seem to have the least problem with allergies, probably because their immune systems are the most environmentally friendly. The combination of A-like and B-like antigens gives Type ABs a double dose of antigens with which to deal with environmental intrusion.

Autoimmune Disorders

AUTOIMMUNE DISORDERS are immune-system breakdowns. Your immune defenses develop what amounts to severe amnesia; they no longer recognize themselves. The result is that they run amok, making autoantibodies, which attack their own tissues. These warlike autoantibodies think they are protecting their turf, but in reality they are destroying their own organs and inciting inflammatory responses. Examples of autoimmune disease include rheumatoid arthritis, lupus nephritis, chronic fatigue syndrome/Epstein-Barr, multiple sclerosis, and amyotrophic lateral sclerosis (Lou Gehrig's disease).

Arthritis
Type Os are the predominant sufferers of the autoimmune disorder arthritis. Type O immune systems are environmentally intolerant, and there are many foods—grains and potatoes among them—whose lectins produce inflammatory reactions in their joints.

My father observed many years ago that Type Os tended to develop a gritty sort of arthritis, a chronic deterioration of the bone cartilage. This is the kind of arthritic condition called osteoarthritis, typically found in the elderly. Type As tend to develop a puffy arthritis, which is the more acute rheumatoid form of the disease—a painful and debilitating breakdown of multiple joints.

In my own practice, most of my patients who suffer from rheumatoid arthritis are Type As. The anomaly of Type As, with their immunologically tolerant systems, developing this form of arthritis may be related to A-specific lectins. Laboratory animals injected with A-specific lectins developed inflammation and joint destruction that was indistinguishable from rheumatoid arthritis.

Just as likely, there is a stress connection. Some studies show that people with rheumatoid arthritis tend to be more high strung and less emotionally hardy. When they have poor coping mechanisms for life stress, the disease progresses more rapidly. This makes some sense in light of what we know about the stress factor, and about Type As who are inherently high strung. Type As with rheumatoid arthritis should certainly incorporate daily relaxation techniques, as well as calming exercises.

Chronic Fatigue Syndrome

In recent years, I have treated many people who suffered from the baffling disease called chronic fatigue syndrome (CFS). The primary symptom is great tiredness. Other more advanced symptoms include painful muscles and joints, persistent sore throats, digestive problems, allergies, and chemical sensitivities.

The most important thing I've learned from my research and clinical work is that CFS may not be an autoimmune disease at all, but rather a liver disease. (I place it in this section because that's where people are accustomed to looking for it.)

Although CFS masquerades as a virus or autoimmune disease, the root cause is more likely a problem of poor metabolism in the liver. In other words, the liver is unable to detoxify chemicals. To my reasoning, only this sort of liver problem could produce immunological effects as well as effects characteristic of other systems, such as digestive or musculoskeletal.

I've found that Type O CFS patients in particular do very well on licorice and potassium supplements, in addition to the Type O Diet. Licorice has many effects in the body, but in the liver it really shines. The bile ducts (where detoxification occurs) become more efficient, with greater protection against chemical damage. This preliminary removal of stress to the liver seems to positively influence the adrenals and blood sugar, increasing energy and producing a feeling of well-being. The blood type–specific exercise activities seem to serve also as a valuable guide to help return to appropriate forms of physical activity. (NOTE: *Please* do not use licorice without a physician's supervision.)

CASE HISTORY: CHRONIC FATIGUE SYNDROME
from Dr. John Prentice, Everett, Washington
Karen, 44: Type B

My colleague Dr. John Prentice tried the Blood Type Plan for the first time on a patient with severe CFS. He wasn't totally convinced it would work, but all efforts to help his very sick patient had failed, and he contacted me when he heard of the work I was doing with CFS patients.

Karen was a tough case. She had suffered terrible fatigue for her entire adult life, and had needed twelve hours of sleep every night since she was a teenager. She would steal naps when she could. For the past seven years her exhaustion prevented her from holding a job. In addition, her neck, shoulders, and back were constantly in pain, and she suffered debilitating headaches. Recently, Karen had started experiencing terrible anxiety attacks, with heart palpitations so severe she would call 911. It felt as if her circulation were shutting down, along with her whole body.

Karen was a wealthy woman, but most of her inheritance was spent on making the rounds to doctors. She had been to more than fifty doctors, both conventional and alternative, before she came to Dr. Prentice.

Dr. Prentice started Karen on a program of strict adherence to the Type B Diet, supplements, and exercise regimen. Both he and Karen were astonished to see that within only a week she had a tremendous increase in energy. Within a few weeks, most of her symptoms were resolved.

Dr. Prentice tells me that today Karen is a new person. "It's like clockwork," he says. "When she eats 'off' her diet, her body reminds her with severe symptoms, so she sticks with it closely." He shared a letter she had written to him: "I have a whole new life. All my symptoms are practically gone and I hold two jobs, having great energy fourteen hours a day consistently. I believe the diet is key to this tremendous change. I am extremely active and feel like nothing can stop me. Thank you so very much!"

Multiple Sclerosis, Lou Gehrig's Disease
Both multiple sclerosis and Lou Gehrig's disease (amyotrophic lateral sclerosis) are seen in very high frequency in Blood Type B. It's an example of the Type B tendency to contract unusual slow-growing viral and neurological disorders. The Type B association may explain why many Jews, with high numbers of Type B blood, suffer from these diseases more than other groups. Some researchers believe that multiple sclerosis and Lou Gehrig's disease are caused by a virus, contracted in youth, that has a B-like appearance. The virus cannot be combatted by the Type B immune system since it can't produce anti-B antibodies. The virus grows slowly and without symptoms until twenty or more years after it has entered the system.

Type ABs also are at risk for these B-like diseases, since their bodies do not produce anti-B antibodies. Type O and Type A seem to be relatively immune by virtue of their strong anti-B antibodies.

CASE HISTORY: AUTOIMMUNE DISORDER
Joan, 55: Type O

Joan, a middle-aged dentist's wife, was a classic example of the ravages of autoimmune disorders. She suffered from severe

symptoms of chronic fatigue/Epstein-Barr, arthritis, and tremendous discomfort caused by gas and bloating. Joan's digestive system was so disrupted that practically everything she ate caused
bouts of diarrhea. By the time she arrived in my office, she had
been struggling with these conditions for more than a year. Needless to say, she was terribly weakened and in great pain. She was
also very discouraged. Since autoimmune disorders can be hard
to pin down, many people (even some physicians) don't believe
chronic fatigue sufferers are really sick. Imagine the humiliation
and frustration of feeling deathly ill but having people tell you it's
all in your head!

Worse still, Joan's doctors had experimented with a number of
drug therapies, including steroids, which made her even sicker
and contributed to her bloating. She had also been told to adopt
a diet high in grains and vegetables, and to limit or eliminate red
meat—exactly the opposite of what this Type O should have
been doing.

As severe as Joan's symptoms were, the treatment was fairly
simple—a detoxification program, the Type O diet, and a regimen of nutritional supplements. Within two weeks, Joan experienced significant improvement. By the six-month mark, she was
feeling "normal" again. To this day, Joan's energy level is good,
her digestion is healthy, and her arthritis flares up only when she
indulges in the rare sandwich or ice cream.

CASE HISTORY: LUPUS
From Dr. Thomas Kruzel, N.D., Gresham, Oregon
Marcia, 30: Type A

My colleague Dr. Kruzel was interested in trying the blood type
treatments, but he was initially skeptical. It was a case of lupus
nephritis that showed him the true value of serotyping for the
treatment of disease.

Marcia, a frail young woman suffering from lupus, was carried
into Dr. Kruzel's office by her brother after being discharged from
the hospital's intensive-care unit. She had suffered kidney failure

from circulating immune complexes related to her disease. Marcia had been on shunt dialysis for several weeks and was scheduled for renal transplantation within the next six months.

Dr. Kruzel took her history and learned that Marcia's diet was very high in dairy, wheat, and red meat—all dangerous foods for a Type A person in her condition. He placed her on a strict vegetarian diet along with hydrotherapy and homeopathic preparations. Within two weeks, Marcia's condition had improved and her need for dialysis had decreased. Remarkably, within a two-month period, Marcia was taken completely off dialysis and her previously scheduled kidney transplant was canceled. Three years later, she is still doing well.

Blood Disorders

IT SHOULD COME as no surprise that blood-related illnesses, such as anemia and clotting disorders, are blood type specific.

Pernicious Anemia

Type As constitute the greatest number of pernicious anemia sufferers, but the condition has nothing to do with the vegetarian Type A Diet. Pernicious anemia is the result of a vitamin B-12 deficiency, and Type As have the most difficulty absorbing B-12 from the foods they eat. Type ABs also have a tendency toward pernicious anemia, although not as great as Type As.

The reason for the deficiency is that the body's use of B-12 requires high levels of stomach acid and the presence of intrinsic factor, a chemical produced by the lining of the stomach that is responsible for B-12's assimilation. Type As and Type ABs have lower levels of intrinsic factor than the other blood types, and they don't produce that much stomach acid. For this reason, most Type As and Type ABs who suffer from pernicious anemia respond best when vitamin B-12 is administered by injection. By eliminating the need for the digestive process to assimilate this vital and potent nutrient, it is made available to the body in a more highly concentrated way. This is a case where dietary solutions alone don't work, although Type As and Type ABs are able to absorb Floradix, a liquid iron and herb supplement.

Type O and Type B tend not to suffer from anemia; they have high acid contents in their stomachs and sufficient levels of intrinsic factor.

CASE HISTORY: ANEMIA
From Jonathan V. Wright, M.D., Kent, Washington
Carol, 35: Type O

The blood type diets have begun to make their way into conventional medicine, as I have shared them with my M.D. colleagues. Dr. Wright was one who successfully used the diet to treat a woman with chronically low blood levels of iron. Carol had tried every available form of iron supplement with no success. Dr. Wright tried a number of other treatments without success. The only thing that worked at all was injectable iron, but it was only a temporary solution. Her iron levels would inevitably drop again.

I had spoken to Dr. Wright on an earlier occasion about my work with lectins and blood types, and he called me for more details. He decided to try the Type O Diet for Carol. After eliminating the incompatible lectins, which may have been damaging her red blood cells, and adhering to a high–animal protein diet, Carol's blood iron levels started to rise, and previously ineffective supplementation started to help. Dr. Wright and I agreed that the agglutination of the intestinal tract by the incompatible food lectins prevented the iron from assimilating.

Clotting Disorders
Type Os face the biggest problems when it comes to blood clotting. Most often, Type Os lack sufficient quantities of the various blood-clotting factors. This can have severe consequences, especially during surgery, or in situations where there is blood loss. Type O women, for example, tend to lose significantly more blood after childbirth than women of other blood types.

Type Os with a history of bleeding disorders and stroke should emphasize foods containing chlorophyll to help modify their clotting factors. Chlorophyll is found in almost all green vegetables, and also can be taken as a supplement.

Type A and Type AB don't suffer clotting disorders, but their thicker blood can work to their disadvantage in other ways. Thicker blood is more likely to deposit plaque in the arteries— one reason why Type A and Type AB are more prone to cardiovascular disease. Type A and Type AB women might have problems with heavy clotting during their menstrual periods if they don't keep their diets under control.

Type Bs tend not to suffer from clotting disorders or thick blood. As long as they follow the Type B Diet, their balanced systems work efficiently.

Cardiovascular Disease

CARDIOVASCULAR DISEASE is epidemic in Western societies, with many factors to blame, including diet, lack of exercise, smoking, and stress.

Is there a connection between your blood type and your susceptibility to cardiovascular disease? When the famous Framingham [Massachusetts] Heart Study examined the connection between blood type and heart disease, it found no clear-cut blood type distinction as to who gets heart disease. It did, however, discover a strong connection between blood type and who survives heart disease. The study found that Type O heart patients between the ages of thirty-nine and seventy-two had a much higher rate of survival than Type A heart patients in the same age group. This was especially true for men between the ages of fifty and fifty-nine.

Although the Framingham Heart Study did not explore this subject in real depth, it does appear that the same factors involved in surviving heart disease also offer some protection against getting it in the first place. Given these factors, clearly there is a greater risk for Type As and Type ABs. Let's examine them.

The most significant factor is cholesterol, the primary causal factor in coronary artery disease. Most of the cholesterol in our bodies is produced in our livers, but there is an enzyme called phosphatase manufactured in the small intestine that is responsible for the absorption of dietary fats. High-alkaline phosphatase levels, which speed the absorption and metabolism of fats, lead to low serum cholesterol levels. Type O blood normally has the highest natural levels of this enzyme. In Type B, Type AB, and Type A, the alkaline phosphatase enzyme is seen in ever-declining levels, with Type B having the highest level after Type O.

Another factor in type Os' high survival rate is blood-clotting factors. As we discussed earlier, Type Os have fewer clotting factors in their blood. This defect in Type O blood may actually work to their advantage, as this essentially thinner blood is less likely to deposit plaque that will clog the arterial flow. On the other hand, Type A, and to a slightly lesser extent, Type AB, have a consistently higher level of serum cholesterol and triglycerides (blood fats) than do Type O and Type B blood.

CASE HISTORY: HEART DISEASE
Wilma, 52: Type O

Wilma was a fifty-two-year-old Lebanese woman with advanced cardiovascular disease. When I first examined her, she had recently come out of the hospital after receiving a balloon angioplasty, a procedure used to treat clogged coronary arteries. She told me that her cholesterol had been over 350 at the time of the original diagnosis (normal is 200 to 220), and three of her arteries had blockages of over 80 percent.

Since Wilma was Type O, her illness was a bit of a surprise, considering that Type Os normally have a lower-than-average incidence of heart disease. She was also quite a bit younger than most women who present with such severe blockages; women tend not to develop heart disease until long after menopause.

(Remember, though, there are always exceptions. Susceptibilities are not certainties!)

Wilma had always eaten the traditional Lebanese diet, including lots of olive oil, fish, and grains, which most doctors feel is beneficial for the circulatory system. However, five years earlier, at the age of forty-seven, she began to experience pain in her neck and arms. Heart disease didn't even occur to her! She assumed the pain was arthritis, and was stunned when her doctor diagnosed her problem as angina pectoris, pain caused from an inadequate blood and oxygen supply to the heart muscle.

After her angioplasty, Wilma's cardiologist advised her to begin taking the cholesterol-lowering drug Mevacor. A well-read health consumer, Wilma worried about long-term problems with drug therapy, and she wanted to try a natural approach before opting for the drug. That's when she came to me.

Since Wilma was Type O, I suggested that she add lean red meat to her diet. In light of her condition, she was understandably nervous about eating foods that are usually restricted in people with high cholesterol or heart disease. She immediately consulted her cardiologist, who was—no surprise—appalled at the idea. Again, he urged her to take Mevacor. But Wilma was serious about avoiding drug therapy, so she decided to follow the Type O Diet for three months and do a cholesterol check at that time.

Wilma confirmed many of my theories about susceptibility to high cholesterol. Often, through heredity or by other mechanisms, people have high levels of cholesterol in their blood in spite of a severely restricted diet. Usually they have some defect in the manipulation of the internal cholesterol metabolism. My suspicion is that when Type Os eat a lot of certain carbohydrates, (usually wheat products), it modifies the effectiveness of their insulin, resulting in its becoming more potent and longer lasting. From the increased insulin activity, the body stores more fat in the tissues and elevates the triglyceride stores.

In addition to advising Wilma to increase the percentage of red meats in her diet, I also helped her find substitutes for the large amounts of wheat she was consuming, and prescribed an extract of hawthorn (an herb used as a tonic for the heart and arteries) and a low dose of the B vitamin, niacin, which helps reduce cholesterol levels.

Wilma was an executive secretary with a stressful job and she did very little exercise. She was intrigued when I described the relationship between stress and physical activity in people with Type O blood, as well as the relationship between stress and heart disease. She had never been a regular exerciser, so hardly knew where to begin. I started her on a walking program to gradually increase her aerobic fitness. After a couple of weeks, Wilma reported that walking was a godsend; she'd never felt better.

Within six months Wilma's cholesterol plummeted, without medication, to 187, where it stabilized. She was elated to have cholesterol in the normal range. It had seemed impossible.

The naturopath intern working in my office was astounded and perplexed. All conventional evidence indicates that people with high cholesterol should avoid red meats, yet Wilma flourished. Blood type was the missing link.

CASE HISTORY: DANGEROUSLY HIGH CHOLESTEROL
John, 23: Type O

John, a recent college graduate, had a skyrocketing cholesterol level, high triglycerides, and high blood sugar. These were very unusual symptoms in a young man—especially since he was Type O. As there was a strong family history of heart disease, naturally his parents were alarmed. After extensive workups at Yale by consulting cardiologists, John was told that his genetic predisposition was so overwhelming that even cholesterol-reducing medication would be useless. In effect, John was told that he was destined to develop coronary artery disease—sooner, rather than later.

In the office, John seemed depressed and lethargic. He complained of severe fatigue. "I used to love to work out," he said, "but now I just don't have the energy." John also suffered from frequent sore throats and swollen glands. His past history revealed mononucleosis and two separate incidences of Lyme disease.

John had been following a vegetarian diet prescribed by his cardiologist for some time. He admitted, however, that he was feeling worse on this diet, not better.

After only a few weeks on the Type O Diet, however, the results were amazing. Within five months, John's serum cholesterol, triglycerides, and blood sugar all dropped to normal levels. A repeat blood profile after three months revealed similar results.

If John continued to follow the Type O Diet, exercise regularly, and take nutritional supplements, there was a good chance that he would beat the odds of his genetic inheritance.

High Blood Pressure

Constantly at work within us is the dynamic force of our beating hearts, rhythmically pumping blood through our bodies. The process is normally so smooth that we rarely think much about it. That's why high blood pressure (or hypertension) is called the silent killer. It's possible to have dangerously high blood pressure and be entirely unaware of it.

When blood pressure is taken, two numbers are read. The systolic reading (the number on top) measures the pressure within the arteries as your heart beats out blood. The diastolic reading (the number on the bottom) measures the pressure present within the arteries as your heart rests between beats.

Normal systolic pressure is 120, and normal diastolic pressure is 80—or 120 over 80 (120/80). High blood pressure (or hypertension) is 140/90 under age forty, and 160/95 over age forty.

Depending on the severity and duration, high blood pressure left untreated opens the door to a host of problems, including heart attacks and strokes.

Little is known about the blood type–related risk factors for hypertension. However, hypertension often occurs in conjunction with heart disease, so Type As and Type ABs should be particularly vigilant.

Hypertension carries the same risk factors as cardiovascular disease. Smokers, diabetics, post-menopausal women, the obese, the sedentary, and people in stressful positions should pay extra attention to the details of their blood type program—especially to the diet and exercise recommendations.

CASE HISTORY: HYPERTENSION
Bill, 54: Type A

Bill was a middle-aged bond trader with high blood pressure. When I first saw him in my office in March 1991, his blood pressure was an almost explosive 150/105 to 135/95. It didn't take me long to find clues to these numbers in his incredibly stressful life, which included a partnership in a high-powered firm and a host of domestic problems. Against his doctor's urging, Bill had discontinued his blood pressure medication because it made him dizzy and constipated. He wanted to try a more natural therapy, but it had to be done immediately.

I placed Bill on a Type A Diet—a huge adjustment for this burly Italian-American. And I immediately began to address Bill's stress with the exercise regimen designed for Type As. He was initially embarrassed about doing yoga and relaxation exercises, but was soon converted when he saw how much calmer and more positive he felt.

At his first visit, Bill also confided that he had a special problem of a different nature. He and his partners were in the process of negotiating their office health plan, and if his hypertension were detected at his insurance physical, his firm would have to pay a much higher premium. Using the stress-reduction techniques, the Type A Diet, and several botanicals, Bill was able to sail through his insurance physical.

Childhood Illnesses

A LARGE NUMBER of the patients who come through my office are children suffering from a host of ailments—from chronic diarrhea to repeated ear infections. Their mothers are usually on the verge of frantic. Some of my most satisfying results have come with children.

Conjunctivitis

Conjunctivitis, commonly called "pink eye," is usually caused by the transmission of the staphylococcus bacteria from one child to another. Type A and Type AB children are more susceptible to conjunctivitis than are Type O or Type B, probably because of their naturally weaker immune systems.

Antibiotic creams or eyedrops are used to treat the condition in the conventional manner. But a soothing and surprising alternative is a freshly cut slice of tomato. (Don't try this with tomato juice!) The freshly cut tomato water contains a lectin that can agglutinate and destroy the staphylococcccus bacteria. The slight acidity of the tomato appears to resemble closely the acidity of the eye's own secretions. Squeezing the watery juice of a fresh tomato on a gauze pad and applying it to the affected eye is also very soothing.

This is one example of how the same lectins in a food that make it dangerous to eat can be highly beneficial to treat an illness. Later, we'll discuss many other examples of the ways in which lectins play a dual role—good cop, bad cop—in our systems. Especially in the war against cancer.

Diarrhea

Diarrhea can be a disturbing and dangerous condition for children. Not only is it debilitating and terribly uncomfortable, but it can lead to severe dehydration, causing weakness and fever.

Most childhood diarrhea is diet related, and here the Blood Type Diets offer very specific guidelines about which foods trigger digestive problems for each blood type.

Type O children often experience mild to moderate diarrhea in reaction to eating dairy products.

Type A and Type AB children are prone to *Giardiasis lamblia*, more commonly known as Montezuma's Revenge, because the parasite mimics A qualities.

Type B children will contract diarrhea if they overindulge in wheat products, or in reaction to eating chicken and corn.

If the diarrhea is caused by food-related intolerance or allergy, your child will often exhibit other symptoms, ranging from dark, puffy circles under the eyes to eczema, psoriasis, or asthma.

Unless diarrhea is the result of a more serious condition such as a parasitic infection, partial intestinal blockage, or inflammation, it usually corrects itself with time. Should your child's stool contain blood or mucus, however, seek immediate medical attention. Acute diarrhea might also be infectious; to protect the rest of your family from contagion, it is best to institute scrupulous standards of cleanliness.

To restore your child's proper balance of fluids during bouts of diarrhea, restrict fruit juice. Instead, feed your child vegetable or meat stocks in soups. Yogurt with active *L. acidophilus* cultures helps maintain the good bacteria in the intestinal tract.

Ear Infections

Perhaps as many as four out of every ten children under the age of six have chronic ear infections. By chronic, I mean five, ten, fifteen, even twenty infections every winter season, one after the other. Most of these children have allergies to both environmental and food-based particles. The best solution is the Blood Type Diet.

The conventional protocol for ear infections is antibiotic therapy. But it obviously fails when there is a chronic infection. If we attack the underlying causes of the problem first instead of trotting out the most currently fashionable nostrum—and by this I mean the ever more sophisticated and newest classes of antibiotics—we have an opportunity to allow the body to mount its own powerful response. For starters, it is helpful to know the blood type susceptibilities.

Children who are Type A and Type AB have greater problems with mucus secretions from improper diet—a factor in ear infections. In Type A children, dairy products are usually the culprit, whereas Type AB may experience sensitivities to corn in addition to milk. In general, these kids are also more likely to have throat and respiratory problems, which can often move into the ears. Because the immune systems of Type A and Type AB children are tolerant of a wider range of bacteria, some of their problems stem from the lack of an aggressive response to the infectious organism. Several studies have shown that ear fluids of children with a history of chronic ear infections lack specific chemicals called complement, which are needed to attack and destroy the bacteria. Another study shows that a serum lectin called Mannose Binding Protein is missing in the ear fluids of children with chronic infections. This lectin apparently binds to mannose sugars on the surface of the bacteria and agglutinates them, allowing for their faster removal. Both of these important immune factors eventually develop in their proper amounts, which may help to explain why the frequency of ear infections gradually lessens as the child ages. In addition to diet, treating Type A and Type AB children with ear infections almost always involves enhancing their immunity. The simplest way to enhance the immunity of any child is to cut down on their intake of sugar. Numerous studies have shown that sugar depresses the immune system, making the body's white blood cells sluggish and disinclined to attack invading organisms.

Naturopaths have for many years made use of a mild herbal immune stimulant, *Echinacea purpurea.* Originally used by Native Americans, echinacea has the extraordinary properties of being both safe and effective in boosting the body's immunity against bacteria and viruses. Since many of the immune functions that echinacea enhances depend on adequate levels of vitamin C, I often prescribe an extract of vitamin C–rich rose hips. In the last three years I have been using an extract of the western larch tree as a sort of super-echinacea. This product originally developed out of the paper-pulping industry and contains much more concentrated active components than you get with echinacea. In my opinion, this product is an exciting new development that has revolutionized my treatment of a variety of immune deficiencies, including ear infections. I'm sure you'll be hearing much more about it in the very near future. (See Appendix F for more details.)

Ear infections are terribly painful for a child, and not too pleasant for the parents, either. Most of these infections are a backup of noxious fluids and gases into the middle ear because of an obstructed connecting pipe, the eustachian tube. This tube can become swollen because of allergic reactions, weakness in the tissues surrounding it, or infections.

Many parents have grown frustrated by the increasing inability of antibiotics to work on ear infections. There is a reason why this happens. A baby's first ear infection is typically treated with a mild antibiotic such as Amoxicillin. With the child's next ear infection, Amoxicillin is given again. Eventually, the ever more resistant infection returns, and Amoxicillin is no longer effective. The escalation phenomenon—the process of using stronger and stronger drugs and ever more invasive treatments—has begun.

When antibiotics no longer work, and the painful infections continue, a myringotomy is performed. This is a process in which tiny tubes called grommets are surgically implanted through the eardrum to increase the drainage of fluid from the middle ear into the throat.

When I treat chronic ear infections, I focus on ways to prevent recurrences. It is useless to try to resolve one episode with a quick dose of antibiotics when you know another ear infection is warming up in the bullpen. Almost always, I find a solution in the diet.

I see many children in my practice, representing all blood types. I've found that any child can contract chronic ear infections if he eats foods that react poorly in his system. I have never seen a case where there wasn't an obvious connection in a child's favorite food.

Type O and Type B children seem to develop ear infections less frequently, and when they do occur, they are usually easier to treat. More often than not, a change in diet is sufficient to eliminate the problem.

In Type B children, the culprit is usually a viral infection that then leads to infection with a bacteria called hemophilus, to which Type B is unusually susceptible. The dietary fix involves restricting tomatoes, corn, and chicken. The lectins in these foods react with the surface of the digestive tract, causing swelling and mucus secretion, which usually carries over to the ears and throat.

My personal feeling is that ear infections can be prevented in Type O children simply by breast-feeding instead of bottle feeding. Breast-feeding for a period of a year or so allows a child's immune system and digestive tract time to develop. Type O kids will also avoid ear infections if they are taken off wheat and dairy products. They're unusually sensitive to these foods at an early age, but their immunity is easily augmented by the use of higher-value proteins such as fish and lean red meats.

Dietary changes are often difficult in households with children who suffer repeated ear infections. Their misery often tempts the anxious parent to let them eat whatever they wish, thinking that it will comfort them. Many of these kids wind up being picky eaters, eating only a very narrow range of foods, and often the very foods that are provoking their illness!

CASE HISTORY: EAR INFECTION
Tony, 7: Type B

Tony was a seven-year-old boy who suffered from repeated ear infections. When his mother first brought him to my office in January 1993, she was frantic. Tony would develop a new ear infection immediately after stopping the antibiotic used to treat his previous infection—at the rate of ten to fifteen per winter season. He had had grommet treatment twice, to no avail. This was a perfect example of a child on the antibiotic treadmill—escalating levels of antibiotics with fewer results.

My initial questions to Tony's mother were about his diet. She was a bit defensive. "Oh, I don't think that's the problem," she told me. "We eat very well—lots of chicken and fish, fruits and vegetables."

I turned to Tony. "What are your favorite foods?" I asked.

"Chicken nuggets," he replied enthusiastically.

"Do you like corn on the cob?"

"Oh, yes!"

"And therein lies the problem," I said to Tony's mother. "Your son is allergic to chicken and corn."

"He is?" She regarded me doubtfully. "How do you know that?"

"Because he's Blood Type B," I replied. I explained the blood type connection and, although Tony's mother was unconvinced, I suggested she feed Tony the Type B Diet for two or three months to see what would happen.

The rest, as they say, is history. Over the next two years Tony did very well, usually developing a single ear infection per season—as opposed to his previous rate of ten to fifteen. These isolated infections were easy to treat either with naturopathic methods, or a gentle low-strength antibiotic.

Hyperactivity and Learning Disabilities

There are a variety of different causes for attention deficit disorders (ADD), and we still need much more information before we can make a conclusive blood type connection. We can, however, gain some insight from our knowledge of how different blood types respond to their environments. For example, my father has observed over thirty-five years of practice that Type O children are happier, healthier, and more alert when they're given the opportunity to exercise to their maximum potential. A Type O child with ADD should be encouraged to exercise as much as possible. This might include additional gym classes, team sports, or gymnastics. Type A and Type AB children, on the other hand, seem to benefit from activities that encourage the development of sensory and tactile skills, such as sculpting or artwork, and from basic relaxation techniques, such as deep breathing. Type B children do well with swimming and calisthenics.

There is some speculation among researchers that ADD is the result of sugar metabolism being out of whack, or allergies to dyes or other chemicals. There is no real conclusion that can be drawn at this point, although I've noticed that ADD kids tend to be incredibly fussy eaters—which suggests a dietary connection.

I recently discovered an interesting connection that might more strongly tie Type O children to ADD. A Type O child was brought to me who suffered from both ADD and mild anemia. I placed him on a high-protein diet and gave him supplements of vitamins B-12 and folic acid, and the anemia cleared up. But his mother also noticed a decided improvement in her child's attention span. I've subsequently treated several Type O ADD children with low doses of these vitamins and have seen improvements ranging from slight to dramatic.

If your child has ADD, talk to a nutrition professional about adding supplements of vitamin B-12 and folic acid, in addition to the Blood Type Diet.

Strep Throat, Mononucleosis, and Mumps

Because the early symptoms of mononucleosis and the symptoms of strep throat are similar, it is often difficult for parents to differentiate between the two. A child with either illness may exhibit one or more of the following symptoms: sore throat, malaise, fever, chills, headache, swollen glands, or swollen tonsils. A blood test and throat culture will be needed to determine which illness is causing the problem.

Strep throat, caused by the streptococcal organism, is a bacterial infection. It often has the additional symptoms of nasal discharge, cough, earaches, white or yellow patches on the back of the throat, and a rash that starts on the neck and chest and spreads to the abdomen and extremities. Diagnosis of strep throat is based on clinical symptoms and a throat culture. The standard treatment includes antibiotics, bed rest, and aspirin and fluids for aches and fever.

Once again, the focus is on treating the immediate infection, not on solving the larger and more long-term health issues. Especially when your child suffers repeat infections, the standard therapy is ineffective.

In general, Type O and Type B children contract strep throat

more often than do Type A and Type AB because of their increased vulnerability to bacterial infections. However, Type O
and Type B also recover more easily and completely. Once the
strep organism gets into the bloodstream of Type A and Type AB,
it settles in and doesn't want to leave. Thus, Type A and Type AB
children will have repeated infections.

There are naturopathic therapies that can help prevent recurrences. I have found that using a mouth rinse made from the
herbs sage and goldenseal is very effective in keeping the throat
and tonsils free from strep. Goldenseal contains a component
called berberine, which has been well studied for its anti-strep
activity. The problem with goldenseal is that it has a distinctly
bitter, weedy taste which kids don't exactly relish. It is sometimes easier to purchase an inexpensive atomizer or spray pump
bottle and just spray the back of your child's throat a couple of
times a day. In addition to the Blood Type Diets, I often use nutritional supplements for immune support, in the form of additional beta-carotene, vitamin C, zinc, and echinacea to help
develop the child's resistance.

With the viral infection mononucleosis, Type O seems to be
more susceptible than Type A, Type B, or Type AB. Antibiotics
are ineffective in the treatment of mononucleosis because it is
caused by a virus, not a bacteria. Bed rest while the fever lasts and
frequent rest intervals during the one- to three-week recovery
period are recommended. Aspirin and adequate fluid intake is
encouraged to decrease fever.

Type B children seem to be more at risk for developing severe
mumps, a viral infection of the salivary glands under the chin and
ears. Like many B-prone illnesses, this one has a neurological
connection. If your child is Type B and/or Rh– (see explanation
in Appendix E, The Blood Type Subgroups) and has the mumps,
be alert for signs of neurologic damage, particularly as manifested
in hearing problems.

Diabetes

THE BLOOD TYPE DIETS can be effective in the treatment of Type I (childhood) diabetes, and in both the treatment and prevention of Type II (adult) diabetes.

Blood Type A and Type B are more prone to Type I diabetes, caused by a lack of insulin, the hormone manufactured by the pancreas responsible for allowing glucose to enter the cells of the body. The cause of insulin deprivation is the destruction of the beta cells of the pancreas, which are the sole cells capable of producing insulin.

Although there is currently no effective natural-treatment alternative for injectable insulin-replacement therapy in Type I diabetics, one important natural remedy to consider using is quercetin, an antioxidant derived from plants. Quercetin has been shown to help prevent many of the complications stemming from lifelong diabetes, such as cataracts, neuropathy, and cardio-vascular problems. Talk with a nutritionist who is skilled in the use of phytochemicals if you plan on using any natural medicine for diabetes; you may have to readjust your insulin dosage.

Type II diabetics typically have high levels of insulin in their bloodstreams, but their tissues lack sensitivity to insulin. This condition develops over time and is usually the result of a poor diet. Type II diabetes is often observed in Type Os who have eaten dairy, wheat, and corn products for many years; and in Type As who eat a lot of meat and dairy foods. Type II diabetics are usually overweight and often have high cholesterol and elevated blood pressure—signs of a lifetime of poor food choices and lack of exercise. In this respect, any blood type can develop Type II diabetes.

The only real treatment for Type II diabetes is diet and exercise. Your Blood Type Diet and exercise regimen will achieve results if you stick to the guidelines. A high-potency vitamin B complex can also help to counter insulin intolerance. Again, check with a physician and nutritionist before using any substance to treat your diabetes. You might have to adjust the dosage of your diabetic medication.

Digestive Illnesses

Constipation

Constipation occurs when the stools are unusually hard or a person's bowel patterns have changed and become less frequent. Most chronic constipation is caused by poor bowel habits and irregular meals, with a diet low in bulk and water content. Some other causes are a habitual use of laxatives, a rushed and stressful daily schedule, and travel that requires abrupt adjustments of eating and sleeping patterns. Lack of physical exercise, acute illness, painful rectal conditions, and some medications also may cause constipation.

Every blood type is susceptible to constipation given the circumstances. Constipation is not so much a disease as a warning flare that something is not right with your digestive system. You'll find most of the clues in your diet.

Are you eating enough foods on your diet that are high in fiber content? Are you drinking enough fluids—in particular, water and juices? Are you exercising regularly?

Many people simply take a laxative when they're constipated. But that doesn't solve the natural systemic causes of constipation. The long-term solution is in the diet. However, Type A, Type B, and Type AB can supplement their diets with fibrous unprocessed bran. Type Os, in addition to eating plenty of the fibrous fruits and vegetables on their diets, can take a supplement of butyrate, a natural bulk-forming agent as a substitute for bran which is not advised for them.

Crohn's Disease and Colitis

These are depleting, enervating diseases that add the elements of uncertainty, pain, blood loss, and suffering to the process of elimination. Many food lectins can cause digestive irritation by attaching to the mucous membranes of the digestive tract. As many of the food lectins are blood type specific, it is possible for each blood type to develop the same problem from different foods.

In Type As and Type ABs, Crohn's disease and colitis often involve a major stress component. If you have Type A or Type AB blood and suffer from inflammatory bowel disease, pay careful attention to your stress patterns and refer to the discussion of stress in your Blood Type Plan.

Type Os tend to develop the more ulcerative form of colitis that causes bleeding with elimination. This is probably due to the lack of adequate clotting factors in their blood. Type As, Type ABs, and Type Bs tend to develop more of a mucous colitis, which is not as bloody. In either case, follow the diet for your blood type. You will be able to avoid many of the food lectins that can aggravate the condition, and you may find your symptoms easing.

CASE HISTORY: IRRITABLE BOWEL SYNDROME
Virginia, 26: Type O

I first examined Virginia, a twenty-six-year-old woman with chronic bowel trouble, three years ago, after she had received extensive treatment from a variety of conventional gastroenterologists. Her problems included chronic irritable bowel syndrome with painful constipation alternating with an unpredictable, almost explosive diarrhea that made it difficult for her to leave the house. She also suffered from fatigue and low-grade chronic anemia. Her previous doctors conducted an enormous amount of testing (to the tune of $27,000!) and could only suggest anti-spasmodic drugs and a daily dose of fiber. Food allergy testing was inconclusive. Virginia was a vegetarian who followed a strict macrobiotic diet, and I immediately detected the foods in her diet that were causing her suffering. The absence of meat in her diet was a primary factor. She also was unable to properly digest the grains and pasta she was eating as a main course.

Since Virginia was Type O, I suggested a high-protein diet, in-

cluding lean red meats, fish and poultry, and fresh fruits and vegetables. As the digestive tract of Type O does not tolerate most
grains very well, I suggested that she avoid whole wheat altogether and severely limit her consumption of other grains.

Initially, Virginia was resistant to the idea of making these dietary changes. She was a vegetarian and she believed that her
current diet was truly healthier. But I urged her to look again.
"How has this diet helped you, Virginia?" I asked. "You seem to
be pretty sick."

Eventually, I convinced her to try it my way for a limited period of time. In eight weeks Virginia returned looking hale and
hardy, with a ruddy complexion. She boasted that her bowel
problems were 90 percent better. Blood tests showed a complete
resolution of her anemia, and she said her energy levels were almost back to normal. A second follow-up visit one month later resulted in Virginia's being discharged from my care, completely
free of bowel problems.

CASE HISTORY: CROHN'S DISEASE
Yehuda, 50: Type O

I first saw Yehuda, a middle-aged Jewish man, in July 1992 for active Crohn's disease. By that point he had already had several
bowel surgeries to remove sections that were obstructing his
small intestine. I put Yehuda on a wheat-free diet, with an emphasis on lean meats and boiled vegetables. I also gave him a
high-powered extract of licorice and the fatty acid butyrate.

Yehuda's compliance was exemplary, a testament to the concerns both he and his family had for his health. For example, his
wife, the daughter of a baker, baked him a special wheat-free
bread. Yehuda took his supplements, including the licorice, very
seriously, as he took everything else.

From the start, Yehuda consistently improved. To this day he
continues to be asymptomatic, although he must still be careful
about using certain grains and dairy products, as they bother his

digestion. He never required additional surgery, even though his gastroenterologist had earlier said it was inevitable.

Case History: Crohn's Disease
Sarah, 35: Type B

Sarah was a thirty-five-year-old woman of eastern European ancestry. She first came to my office in June 1993 for treatment of Crohn's disease. She had already had several surgeries to remove scarred tissue from the bowel, was anemic, and suffered from chronic diarrhea.

I prescribed a basic Type B diet, instructing that Sarah remove chicken and other lectin-containing foods specific for Type B. I also used supplemental licorice and fatty acids as part of her protocol.

Sarah was very cooperative. Within four months, most of her digestive symptoms, including the diarrhea, were eliminated. As she wanted to have more children, Sarah recently had surgery to remove scar tissue from her bowel that had attached to her uterus. Her surgeon told her that there was no sign of active Crohn's disease anywhere in her abdominal cavity.

Food Poisoning

Anyone can get food poisoning. But certain blood types are naturally more susceptible because of their tendency toward a weakened immune system. In particular, Type A and Type AB are more likely to fall prey to salmonella food poisoning, which is usually the result of leaving food uncovered and unrefrigerated for long periods of time. Furthermore, the bacteria will be harder for Type A and Type AB to get rid of once they've found a home in their systems.

Type Bs, who are generally more susceptible to inflammatory diseases, are more likely to be severely affected when they eat food that is contaminated with the shigella organism, a bacteria found on plants that causes dysentery.

Gastritis

Many people confuse gastritis with ulcers, but it is exactly the opposite. Ulcers are produced by hyperacidity—more common for Type O and Type B. Gastritis is caused by very low stomach acid content—common for Type A and Type AB. Gastritis occurs when the stomach acid gets so low that it no longer functions as a microbial barrier. Without adequate levels of acid, microbes will live in the stomach and cause serious inflammation.

The best course of action that Type A and Type AB can take is to stress the more acidic food choices in their Blood Type Diets.

Stomach and Duodenal Ulcers

It has been known since the early 1950s that peptic ulcer of the stomach is more common in Blood Type O, with the highest occurrence in Type O non-secretors. Type Os also have a higher rate of bleeding and perforation, which was not shown to be different between secretors and non-secretors. One reason is that Type Os have higher stomach-acid levels and an ulcer-producing enzyme called pepsinogen.

More recent research has uncovered another reason why Type Os are prone to ulcers. In December 1993, researchers at Washington University School of Medicine in St. Louis reported in the *Journal of Science* that people with Type O blood are a favorite target for the bacteria now known to cause ulcers. This bacteria, *H. pylori*, was found to be able to attach itself to the Type O antigen lining the stomach, and then work its way into the lining. As we've seen, the Type O antigen is the sugar fucose. The researchers found an inhibitor in breast milk, which apparently blocked the attachment of the bacteria to the stomach surface. No doubt this is one of the many fucose sugars found in human breast milk.

The common seaweed bladder wrack is an inhibitor of *H. pylori*. The content of fucose in bladder wrack is so great that it factors into its Latin name—*Fucus vesiculosis*. If you are Type O and suffer from ulcers or want to prevent them, using bladder wrack will make the ulcer-causing bacteria, *H. pylori*, slide off your stomach lining.

CASE HISTORY: CHRONIC STOMACH ULCERS
Peter, 34: Type O

I first met Peter in April 1992. He had suffered from stomach ulcers since he was a child, and had used every conventional ulcer medication available, with little result. I began by prescribing the basic high-protein Type O Diet, stressing that he avoid the whole wheat products that had always been a major part of his diet. I also prescribed a supplement of bladder wrack, and a combination medicine of licorice and bismuth.

Within six weeks Peter had made considerable progress. On a follow-up visit to his gastroenterologist, he was "scoped" and heard the encouraging news that 60 percent of his stomach lining now appeared normal. A second examination in June 1993 showed complete resolution of Peter's stomach ulcers.

Infections

MANY BACTERIA prefer specific blood types. In fact, one study showed that over 50 percent of 282 bacteria carried antigens of one blood type or another.

It has been observed that viral infections in general seem to be more frequent in Type Os because they do not possess any antigens. These infections are less frequent and milder in Type A, Type B and Type AB.

Acquired Immune Deficiency Syndrome (AIDS)

I have treated many people who were HIV positive or had full-blown AIDS, and I have yet to find a clear-cut connection between blood type and susceptibility to HIV. Having said that, let's look at how the information in this book can be used to help people hold their own against the virus.

While all the blood types appear to be equally susceptible to AIDS, given the exposure, there are variations in their suscepti-

bility to the opportunistic infections (such as pneumonia and tuberculosis) that their weakened immune systems fall prey to.

If you are HIV positive or have AIDS, modify your diet to en-
compass the suggestions that are specific to your blood type. For
example, if you are Type O, begin to increase the amount of animal proteins in your diet and develop a physical training program.
Following the blood type program will help to fully mobilize and
optimize your immune functions by stressing the highest-value
foods for your particular needs. Be careful to limit your fat intake,
choosing lean cuts of meat, because bowel parasites, common in
people with AIDS, interfere with fat digestion and lead to diarrhea. Also avoid foods such as wheat that contain lectins that
could further compromise your immune system and bloodstream.

Since many of the opportunistic infections cause nausea, diarrhea, and mouth sores, AIDS is often a wasting disease. Type As
will need to work a little harder to be sure that their calorie intake
is high, since many Type A foods are calorically low. Rigorously
eliminate any foods, such as meat or dairy, that can cause digestive problems. Your immune system is already naturally sensitive;
don't give the lectins a chance to get in and weaken you further.
Meanwhile, increase your portions of "good" Type A foods, such
as tofu and seafood.

Type Bs should avoid the obvious problem foods, such as
chicken, corn, and buckwheat. But you should also eliminate
nuts, which are hard to digest, and reduce the amount of wheat
products in your diet. If you are lactose intolerant, avoid dairy
foods; even if you're not, dairy can be a digestive irritant for im-
mune-compromised Type Bs. This is a case where the disease is
contraindicative of the favored food.

Type ABs should limit their intake of lectin-rich beans and
legumes, and eliminate nuts from their diets. Your primary protein source should be fish, and there is a wide variety available to
Type ABs. Occasional servings of meat and dairy are okay, but
watch the fat. And limit your wheat consumption.

In general, whatever your blood type, you want to avoid
lectins that could damage the cells of your immune system and

bloodstream. These cells cannot be as easily replaced, the way they are in a healthy body. This cell-sparing aspect of the Blood Type Diets makes them invaluable to the person with AIDS who has anemia or low T-helper cells.

The Blood Type Diets add a powerful rook to your chessboard, helping preserve your precious immune cells from unnecessary damage. This can be a critical difference, especially as there are no really successful treatments for HIV infection.

CASE HISTORY: AIDS
Arnold, 46: Type AB

Arnold was a middle-aged businessman with AIDS. He was married and believed he had been infected with HIV twelve years earlier. When I first saw him, Arnold's T-cell count, the barometer of the virus's destruction, was 6, with normal being 650 to 1,700. He had a skin condition called molluscum, which is often seen in end-stage AIDS, and he was painfully thin from months of diarrhea and nausea.

Arnold decided to come to a naturopath as a desperate, last-ditch effort to stay alive. I could see in his face that he didn't really believe this would work, either, and I couldn't promise him dramatic results because I didn't really know what to expect.

My first goal was to prevent any lectins that were toxic to the Type AB immune system from entering his body. Along with that, it was urgent that I halt Arnold's wasting so he would be strong enough to fight the infection.

I began by tailoring the Type AB Diet to the special needs raised by AIDS. This included the elimination of all poultry except turkey, the introduction of low-fat organic meats, seafood several times a week, rice, lots of vegetables and fruit. I reduced most of the beans and legumes, and eliminated butter, cream, processed cheese, corn, and buckwheat. In addition, I prescribed immune-boosting herbs, in tablet and tea form, including alfalfa, burdock, echinacea, ginseng, and ginger.

Within three months, Arnold's molluscum cleared up and he

was back in the gym. To this day he continues to be asymptomatic, even though his T-cells have not increased. He works and leads a fairly active life. The physicians at the infectious disease center of his hospital are amazed. This is a man without an immune system!

CASE HISTORY: AIDS
Susan, 27: Type O

After learning that her husband was HIV-positive, Susan was tested. She was frantic when she learned that she had HIV. Lab tests revealed a very low T-cell count. Susan begged me to help her; she didn't want to die, and she was afraid to take AZT or any other drug specified for HIV.

We began with a Type O Diet, along with nutritional supplements and regular exercise, instructing Susan to follow the program closely.

A few months later, Susan called to report that her T-cell count was in the 800s (normal is 500 to 1700). She has been symptom free ever since.

Since there is at present no cure for HIV or AIDS, we can't gauge how long Susan will continue to do well. But I believe that the more we discover about the mysteries of the immune system, the closer we'll come to making AIDS a disease to live with, rather than a disease to die from.

Bronchitis and Pneumonia
In general, type A and type AB have more bronchial infections than Type O and Type B. This may result from improper diets that produce excessive mucus in their respiratory passages. This mucus facilitates the growth of blood type–mimicking bacteria, such as the A-like pneumococcus bacteria in Type A and Type AB, and the B-like hemophilus bacteria in Type B and Type AB. (Since Type AB has both A-like and B-like characteristics, the risk is double.)

The Blood Type Diets seem to substantially reduce the incidences of bronchitis and pneumonia for all blood types. However, we are just beginning to discover some other blood type connections that are not so easily remedied. For example, it appears that Type A children born to Type A fathers and Type O mothers die more frequently of broncho-pneumonia in early life. It is thought that some form of sensitization occurs at birth between the Type A infant and the mother's anti-A antibodies that inhibits the infant's ability to fight the pneumococcus bacteria. There is no solid data yet to confirm the reason this occurs, but information of this kind can spark research interest in a potential vaccine. We'll have to gather much more data before we can make a valid scientific conclusion.

Candidiasis (Common Yeast Infection)

Although the candidiasis organism shows no preference for blood type, I have noticed that Type A and Type AB have a tougher time eradicating a severe yeast overgrowth once the organism finds a home in their tolerant systems. Candidiasis becomes like the unwanted guest who won't leave. Type A and Type AB also develop more yeast infections after antibiotic usage, which makes sense, because antibiotics destroy their already weakened defense systems.

Type Os, on the other hand, develop more of an allergic-type hypersensitivity to the candidiasis organism, especially if they eat too many grains. This has been the basis of a theory called the yeast syndrome and a variety of candida diets. These diets stress high protein intake and the avoidance of grains, but they tend to be generalized across blood types, when it is only Type Os who appear to have this yeast sensitivity. If you're Type A or Type AB, yeast avoidance won't do anything to prevent yeast infections, and you'll only further compromise your immune system.

In general, Type Bs are less prone to this organism, as long as they follow the Type B Diet. If you are a Type B who has a history of candidiasis, cut down on your wheat consumption.

Cholera

A report from Peru recently published in the *Lancet* attributed the severity of a recent epidemic of cholera, an infection characterized by extreme diarrhea with severe fluid and mineral depletion, to the high incidence of Type Os in the Peruvian population. Historically, the susceptibility of Type Os to cholera was probably responsible for the decimation of the population of many of the ancient cities, leaving as survivors the more cholera-resistant Type As.

Common Cold and Flu

There are hundreds of different strains of cold virus, and it would be impossible to see blood type specificity in all of them. However, studies of British military recruits showed a slightly lower overall incidence of cold viruses in recruits who were Type A, which is consistent with our findings that Blood Type A was developed to resist these common viruses. Viruses also have less impact on Type AB. The A antigen, carried by both Type A and Type AB, blocks the attachment of various strains of flu to the membranes of the throat and respiratory passages.

Influenza, a more serious virus, also strikes Type O and Type B in preference to Type A and Type AB. In its early stages, influenza may have many of the symptoms of a common cold. However, the flu causes dehydration, muscle pains, and serious weakness.

The symptoms of a common cold or flu are miserable, but they are actually a sign that your immune system is trying hard to fight off the offending virus. While your immune system is doing its job, there are measures you can take that will make coexistence on the battlefield more comfortable:

1. Maintain general good health with adequate rest and exercise, along with learning to cope with the stresses of life. Stress is a major factor in the depletion of immune system resources. This may protect you from frequent

infections and may even shorten the duration of the colds and flus you do get.

2. Follow the basic dietary protocol for your blood type. It will optimize your immune response and help shorten the course of your cold or flu.

3. Take vitamin C (250 to 500 mg), or increase the sources of vitamin C in your diet. Many people feel that taking small doses of the herb echinacea helps prevent colds, or at least helps shorten their duration.

4. Increase the humidity in your room with a vaporizer or humidifier to prevent a dry throat and nasal tissue.

5. If your throat is sore, gargle with salt water. One-half teaspoon of ordinary table salt and a tall glass of comfortably warm water provides a soothing and cleansing rinse. Another good gargle, especially if you are prone to tonsilitis, is a tea of equal parts goldenseal root *(Hydrastis canadensis)* and sage. Gargle with this mixture every few hours.

6. If your nose is runny or stuffy, use an antihistamine to reduce the reaction of tissues to the infecting virus and relieve nasal congestion. Be especially careful with Ephedra-type antihistamines, such as those found in health food stores and in some over-the-counter decongestants. These can raise the blood pressure, keep you awake at night, and complicate prostate problems in men.

7. Antibiotics are not effective against viruses, so if someone offers you leftover antibiotics, or if you have some around the house, don't take them.

Plague, Typhoid, Smallpox, and Malaria

Known during the Middle Ages as the Black Death, plague is a bacterial infection carried largely by rodents. Blood Type O people are more susceptible to plague. Although plague is rare in industrialized societies, it continues to be a problem in Third

World countries. A recent report by the World Health Organization warned that we may be facing a crisis in the appearance of plague and other infectious diseases as a result of overuse of antibiotics and other medicines, human settlement of previously uninhabited areas, international travel, and poverty. The fact that Western societies rarely encounter these diseases should not make us feel immune to their social, economic, cultural and human cost. And occasionally an outbreak does occur in the West, as happened in Seattle in the early 1980s, when people ate tainted tofu that had not been pasteurized. Commercial tofu in sealed packaging should not be a cause for concern.

Smallpox has been officially eradicated through extensive worldwide immunization, although its course has probably influenced world history to a largely unappreciated degree. Blood Type O is especially susceptible to smallpox, which probably explains why the Native American population was decimated by the disease when it first came into contact with the Type A and B European settlers who carried it. Native Americans are almost 100 percent Type O.

Typhoid, a common infection in areas of diminished hygiene or in times of war, usually infects the blood and the digestive tract. Type O is also most susceptible to typhoid infection. Typhoid also shows a connection to the Rh blood groups, being found more frequently in Rh− individuals.

It is claimed that the anopheles mosquito, which carries malaria, tends to bite Type B and Type O in preference to Type A and Type AB, although the common mosquito seems to prefer Type A and Type AB. Malaria is, again, an unfamiliar disease to the Western world, yet its global impact is tremendous. According to the World Health Organization, more than 2.1 million people contract malaria every year.

Polio and Viral Meningitis
Polio, a viral infection of the nervous system, shows a higher frequency in Type B, which is more susceptible to virally sparked nervous system disorders. Polio was epidemic and caused most

cases of juvenile paralysis before the development of the Salk and Sabin vaccines.

Viral meningitis, an increasingly frequent and serious infection of the nervous system, is significantly more common in Type O than in other blood types, probably because of the Type O weakness against aggressive infections. Be alert to symptoms of fatigue, high fever, and a characteristic of meningitis called nuchal rigidity, a stiffness in the muscles of the neck.

Sinus Infections

Type O and Type B are also typically more prone to chronic sinus infections. Very often, their physicians will prescribe an almost continuous supply of antibiotics, which banish the problem temporarily. But the sinus infections inevitably return, prompting the use of more antibiotics and, finally, surgery.

I have found that the herb collinsonia (stone root), which is used to treat swelling problems, such as varicose veins, also helps sinusitis—perhaps because chronic sinusitis is a sort of hemorrhoid or varicose vein of the head. When I prescribe this herb to my patients with chronic sinusitis, the results are often astounding. Many of these patients no longer need antibiotics to treat their infections because the collinsonia removed the cause of the problem—swelling of the sinus tissue. If you have sinus problems, you may wish to try this herb. Collinsonia is not easy to find, but many of the larger health food stores carry it in a liquid tincture form. A typical dose is twenty to twenty-five drops in warm water taken orally two or three times daily. No need to worry about toxicity; this is a safe herb.

Occasionally a Type A or Type AB will develop sinusitis, although this is almost always the result of a highly mucus-forming diet. Sinusitis in Type As usually responds well to diet changes alone.

Parasites
(Amoebic Dysentery, Giardia,
Tapeworm, and Ascaris)

Given enough of a head start, parasites can live fairly well in anyone's digestive tract. By and large, however, they seem to have a
special preference for Type A and Type AB digestive tracts, usually mimicking the Type A blood antigen to avoid detection. For
example, the common amoeba parasite shows a preference for
Type A and Type AB. In addition, it appears that Type A and
Type AB are more prone to complications should amoebic cysts
lodge in the liver. Type A and Type AB with amoebic dysentery
should adopt strong measures to deal with the infection before it
has a chance to migrate farther into their bodies.

Blood Type A and Type AB are also sitting ducks for a common water contaminant, the parasite *Giardia lamblia*, cause of the
condition famously known as Montezuma's Revenge. This clever
parasite mimics the appearance of Type A, which allows it entry
into the Type A and Type AB immune systems, then quickly into
the intestines. Type A and Type AB travelers should equip themselves with the herb goldenseal or Pepto Bismol to help stave off
infection. Type As and Type ABs who drink well water should
also be on the alert for the *Giardia lamblia* parasite.

Many of the parasitic worms, such as the tapeworm and the as-
caris parasite, have a resemblance to Type A and Type B, and are
found in greater frequency in people with these blood types. Because Type AB carries a double A-like, B-like characteristic, Type
ABs are particularly susceptible.

I have used an herb called *Artemesia annua* (Chinese worm-
wood) to treat parasites with notable success. Ask your naturopathic physician about this herb.

Tuberculosis and Sarcoidosis

Once considered almost completely eradicated from Western industrialized society, tuberculosis has now become more common.
This is largely due to the high incidence of the disease among
people with AIDS and the homeless. An opportunistic infection,

tuberculosis thrives in immune systems weakened by poor hygiene and chronic disease. Tuberculosis of the lungs (pulmonary tuberculosis) is more common in Type O, whereas tuberculosis in other parts of the body shows a higher frequency in Type A. Sarcoidosis, or sarcoid, is an inflammatory condition of the lungs and connective tissue that may actually be a form of immune reaction to tuberculosis. It was once thought to be much more common in African-Americans versus the general population, but in recent times it is being diagnosed more frequently in Caucasians, especially women. It shows a higher frequency in Type A over Type O. Rh– individuals seem to be more susceptible to both tuberculosis and sarcoidosis.

Syphilis and Urinary Tract Infections

Blood Type A seems to be more susceptible to the venereal disease syphilis, and often contracts a more virulent strain. This is yet another reason to practice safe sex, especially if you are Type A.

There is good evidence that if you are Type B or Type AB, you are more susceptible to recurrent bladder infections (cystitis). That's because the most common bacteria-producing infections, such as *E. coli*, pseudomonas, and klebsiella, possess a B-like appearance, and Type B and Type AB produce no anti-B antibodies.

Type Bs also have higher rates of kidney infections, such as pyelonephritis. This is especially true of Type B non-secretors. If you are Type B and suffer from recurrent urinary problems, try to drink one or two glasses of a mixture of cranberry and pineapple juice every day.

Liver Disease

Alcoholic-Related Liver Disease

Alcoholism affects many bodily systems, but perhaps its most dramatic impact is on the liver. The 20 percent of the population who are non-secretors (see Appendix E) seem to be the most prone to alcoholism, but their susceptibility has little to do with secretor status. In an unfortunate and possibly random cellular twist, the gene that determines whether you're a non-secretor is located on the same part of the DNA as the gene for alcoholism. My patients who type as non-secretors almost always have an extensive family history of alcoholism.

Oddly enough, it is also non-secretors who seem to derive the most benefit to their hearts from a moderate intake of alcohol. A Danish study showing non-secretors to be at higher risk for ischemic heart disease (a lack of blood flow into the arteries) theorized that a moderate consumption of alcohol altered the rate of insulin flow, slowing the accumulation of fats in the blood vessels. This conflicting message is hard to decipher.

The answer is probably that decisions about the role of alcohol should be made on an individual basis and with consideration of your blood type. Due to the effects of alcohol on the digestive and immune systems, none of the blood type diets allow hard liquor.

It is also clear that alcoholism has a major stress component. A Japanese research team discovered that a greater number of Blood Type As than Type Os or Type Bs received treatment for alcoholism. It is thought that Type As may have a predilection for seeking relaxation from stress by the ingestion of inhibition-releasing chemicals. It is certainly well documented that man has a long history of using intoxicants for pleasure, for pain, for transport to other realms, and for medicine.

Only about 3 percent of the alcohol you consume passes through your body and is excreted. The rest is metabolized by the liver and processed in the stomach and small intestines. Over time, with heavy and regular consumption, the liver begins to deteriorate. The end result can be cirrhosis of the liver, severe malnutrition from malabsorption of foods, and ultimately death.

Gallstones, Cirrhosis, and Jaundice

Of course, not all liver disease is linked to alcohol. Infections, allergies, and metabolic disorders all can cause liver damage. For example, jaundice, or yellowing of the skin, is often seen in people with hepatitis, and gallstones have been linked to obesity. Cirrhosis can be caused by infections, diseases of the bile ducts, or other illnesses that affect the liver.

For reasons we do not fully understand, Type As, Type Bs, and Type ABs tend to have higher levels of gallstones, diseases of the bile ducts, jaundice, and cirrhosis of the liver than Type Os, with Type As having the highest levels. Type As are also reported to be more susceptible to pancreatic tumors.

Liver Flukes and Other Tropical Infections

Common tropical infections of the liver causing fibrosis or scarring appear to a marked degree more frequently in Type As—and to a lesser extent in Type B and Type AB. Type O, which may have developed anti-A and anti-B antibodies as an early protection against these parasites, is relatively immune to them.

My office has successfully treated many cases of liver disease using many of the herbal compounds discussed in chapter 10. In most cases, the patients who develop liver disease are Blood Type A or Type B, non-secretors.

CASE HISTORY: LIVER DISEASE
Gerard, 38: Type B

Gerard was a thirty-eight-year-old man with a history of sclerosing cholangitis, an inflammatory condition of the liver's bile ducts, causing scarring. Usually this condition leads to the necessity of a liver transplant. When I first saw Gerard in July 1994, he was jaundiced and had horrible pruritis (itching) from deposits of bilirubin, a bile pigment, in his skin. Because of this condition, his cholesterol was also elevated (325). Gerard's serum bile acids were over 2,000 (normal is under 100), he had a bilirubin level of 4.1 (normal is under 1) and all his liver enzymes were sharply elevated, indicating extensive damage to his liver tissue. Gerard was a pretty sharp guy, who knew what his chances were, and frankly, he was preparing to die.

I started Gerard on the basic Type B Diet and a botanical pro-tocol of liver-specific antioxidants. These are antioxidants that preferentially deposit in the liver instead of in other organs. Ger-ard did very well in the intervening year, having only one flare-up of his itching and jaundice.

Recently Gerard underwent surgery to remove his gallblad-der. After the surgeon examined his liver and major bile ducts, she told him that they looked normal, although the tissue around his bile ducts was a little thinner than usual.

CASE HISTORY: CIRRHOSIS
Estel, 67: Type A

Estel was sixty-seven-year-old woman who first came to my office in October 1991 for an inflammatory condition of the liver called primary biliary cirrhosis, which results in destruction of the liver. Most cases eventually go on to a liver transplant.

Estel admitted that she was once a heavy drinker, but no longer. Her condition was probably linked to lifetime alcohol consumption. Estel may not have even been an alcoholic in the strictest sense. Three or four drinks a day, every day, for forty years can lead to cirrhosis.

Estel's liver enzymes were markedly elevated: the alkaline phosphatase, for example, was in the high 800s. Normal is under 60. Since she was a Type A non-secretor, I immediately put her on the Type A Diet and a protocol of liver-specific antioxidants. Estel began to show results almost immediately, and her condi-tion continued to improve.

By September 1992, almost a year after her first visit, Estel's alkaline phosphatase had dropped to 500.

Although her liver has shown no signs of further deterioration since that time, Estel developed swelling of the veins around her esophagus, a common condition in people with liver disease, which was treated successfully. She continues to do well and shows no sign of requiring liver transplantation.

CASE HISTORY: LIVER DETERIORATION
Sandra, 70: Type A

Sandra arrived in my office in January 1993, suffering from a difficult-to-determine liver condition. All of her liver enzymes were elevated, and she also had a condition called ascites, an extensive amount of fluid being retained in her abdomen. Ascites is common in many cases of advanced liver failure. Sandra's internist was not treating her liver deterioration, probably expecting her to eventually require a transplant. He was prescribing diuretics to help remove the fluid from her abdomen, but the diuretics were causing her to lose large amounts of potassium, which probably accounted for her overwhelming fatigue.

I prescribed the Type A Diet with liver-specific botanicals. Within four months, all evidence of Sandra's fluid retention disappeared, and her liver enzymes returned to normal. Sandra was initially quite anemic—a hematocrit of 27.1 where normal for a woman is over 38. By February 1994 her hematocrit had risen to 40.8. She continues to be asymptomatic.

Skin Disorders

To DATE, there is little blood type–specific information available on skin disorders. We do know, however, that conditions such as dermatitis and psoriasis usually result from allergic chemicals acting within the blood. It is worth noting again that many of the common food lectins specific for one blood type or another can interact with the blood and digestive tissues, causing the liberation of histamines and other inflammatory chemicals.

Allergic skin reactions to chemicals or abrasives show the highest incidences in Type A and Type AB. Psoriasis is found more frequently in Type Os. My own experience is that many Type Os who develop psoriasis are eating diets too high in grains or dairy products.

CASE HISTORY: PSORIASIS
From Anne Marie Lambert, N.D., Honolulu, Hawaii
Mariel, 66: Type O

My colleague Dr. Lambert used my blood type protocol to treat a complicated case of psoriasis in an older woman.

Mariel went to see Dr. Lambert in March 1994. Her symptoms included severe shortness of breath, difficulty walking, with limited range of motion in all joints, psoriasis lesions covering 70 percent of her skin surface, and burning pain throughout her body, especially in her muscles and joints. Her medical history was a catalog of constant medical problems: vaginal/bladder/bowel repairs (1944–45), appendectomy (1949), hysterectomy (1974), history of ovarian cysts, psoriasis (1978), hospitalization for pneumonia (1987), psoriatic arthritis (1991), and osteoporosis (1992).

Mariel told Dr. Lambert that her typical diet was high in dairy, wheat, corn, nuts and processed foods, with a high sugar and fat content. She said that she craved sweets, nuts, and bananas. This was a terrible diet for almost anyone, but it was anathema to someone of Mariel's blood type.

Dr. Lambert immediately started Mariel on a moderated Type O Diet, which initially excluded red meat and nuts, with additional vitamins and minerals. Within two months, there was a marked decrease in swelling of Mariel's joints, improved breathing, and her psoriatic lesions were healing. By June, Mariel's psoriasis covered only 20 percent of her body, and the lesions were nearly healed. There was a marked improvement in her breathing, her pain had lessened by half, and the range of motion in her joints continued to improve. By July, Mariel's psoriasis was no longer evident, there was only slight swelling in the joint spaces, and her breathing was no longer labored.

At a follow-up visit to Dr. Lambert on October 10, 1994, Mariel's breathing had improved, and she had no new lesions on her skin.

Mariel had been to numerous medical professionals since she became ill. She had tried all types of conventional as well as alternative therapies, including food plans specifically designed for psoriatic arthritis and asthma. Although these diets were well intended, none of them was specifically tailored to ensure compatibility with Mariel's blood. The Type O Diet was able to provide nutrition without causing health problems from foods that were incompatible with Mariel's blood. With the exception of some minor pain relief from Chinese herbs, none of the other treatments had been successful. Mariel considered her progress a miracle!

Women/Reproduction

Pregnancy and Infertility

Many of the disorders related to pregnancy result from some form of blood type incompatibility—either between the mother and the fetus, or between the mother and the father. Unfortunately, we have only initial studies on this phenomenon, and have little idea about its ultimate implications. I suggest that you read this section in the spirit of information gathering, not hysteria. Sometimes a little bit of knowledge can be dangerous unless you keep it in perspective.

TOXEMIA OF PREGNANCY

As early as 1905 it was proposed that some form of blood type sensitization resulted in pregnancy toxemia—a poisoning of the blood that can occur in late pregnancy and cause grave illness and even death. In a later study, an excess of Type O women were found to suffer from toxemia, resulting possibly from a reaction to a Type A or Type B fetus.

BIRTH DEFECTS

Blood type incompatibility, which may occur between a Type O mother and a Type A father, has been implicated in several common birth defects, including hydatiform mole, choriocarcinoma, spinal bifida, and anencephaly. Several studies imply that these disorders appear to be maternal ABO incompatibility with fetal nervous and blood tissue.

Hemolytic Disease of the Newborn

Hemolytic (blood-destroying) disease of the newborn is the primary condition related to the positive/negative aspect of your blood (described in Appendix E). It is a condition that afflicts only the offspring of Rh– women, so if you are O, A, B, or AB positive, it doesn't concern you.

Some fifty years ago, researchers discovered that Rh– women who were missing an antigen and who were carrying Rh+ babies had a unique situation. The Rh+ babies carried the Rh antigen on their blood cells. As is not the case with the major blood type system where the antibodies to other blood types develop from birth, Rh– people do not make an antibody to the Rh antigen unless they are first sensitized. This sensitization usually occurs when blood is exchanged between the mother and infant during birth, so the mother's immune system does not have enough time to react to the first baby, and that baby suffers no consequences. However, should a subsequent conception result in another Rh+ baby, the mother, now sensitized, will produce antibodies to the baby's blood type, potentially causing birth defects and even infant death. Fortunately, there is a vaccine for this condition which is given to Rh– women after the birth of their first child, and after every subsequent birth. It shouldn't arise as a problem, but it's best to know your Rh status so you can be certain that the vaccine is administered.

Infertility and Habitual Miscarriage

For forty years, scientists have been studying the reasons why childlessness seems more common among Type A, Type B, and Type AB women than Type O women. Many researchers have suggested that infertility and habitual abortion may be the result of antibodies in a woman's vaginal secretions reacting with blood type antigens on her husband's sperm. A 1975 study of 288 miscarried fetuses showed a predominance of Type A, Type B and Type AB fetuses, which may have been the result of incompatibility with Type O mothers and their anti-A and anti-B antibodies.

A large sample of families showed that the rate of miscarriages were highest when the mother and father were ABO incompatible, as with a Type O mother and a Type A father. In Caucasian and African mothers, Type B fetuses incompatible with the mother's Type O or Type A blood were more frequently found among miscarriages.

This link to infertility is not yet fully established. In my own practice, I find that there are many reasons for fertility problems, including food allergies, poor diet, obesity, and stress.

CASE HISTORY: REPEATED MISCARRIAGE
Lana, 42: Type A

Lana came to my office in September 1993 after a long history of repeated miscarriages. She told me she'd heard about me from someone she had been talking with in the waiting room of her fertility doctor. Lana was desperate. In the previous ten years she'd had over twenty miscarriages, and she was just about to give up on trying to start a family. I suggested that she try the Blood Type A Diet. For the next year, Lana followed the Blood Type Diet assiduously, also taking several botanical preparations to strengthen the muscular tone of her uterus. At the end of the year, she became pregnant. She was thrilled, but also very nervous. Now, in addition to her previous miscarriages, Lana was worried about her age and the possibility of the fetus having Down's syndrome. Her obstetrician recommended amniocentesis, which is common for women over age forty, but I advised against it because the procedure carries a risk of miscarriage. After talking with her husband, Lana decided to forgo the amniocentesis, accepting the possibility of a birth defect. In January 1995, she delivered a perfectly healthy baby boy.

CASE HISTORY: INFERTILITY
Nieves, 44: Type B

Nieves, a forty-four-year-old South American massage therapist, first came to see me in 1991 for a variety of digestive problems. Within one year of beginning the Type B Diet, most of her digestive complaints were resolved.

One day Nieves shyly announced to me that she was pregnant. Although she had not told me before, she now said that she and her husband had tried for many years to conceive a child, but had finally given up hope. She believed that the Type B Diet was responsible for restoring her fertility. Approximately nine months later, Nieves delivered a healthy baby girl. She was named Nasha, meaning "gift from God."

NOTE: SEX RATIOS
In both European and non-European populations, the rate of male offspring is higher in Type O babies born to Type O mothers. This is also true if both the baby and mother are Type B. The opposite is true of Type A babies born to Type A mothers, where female offspring are more frequent.

Menopause and Menstrual Problems
Menopause affects every midlife woman regardless of her blood type. A decrease in estrogen and progesterone, the two basic female hormones, causes profound mental and physical problems for many women, including hot flashes, loss of libido, depression, hair loss, and skin changes.

The decline in female hormones also creates a risk for cardiovascular disease, as it appears that estrogen provides protection to the heart and lowers cholesterol levels. Osteoporosis, a thinning of the bones that leads to frailty and even death, is another outcome of estrogen deficiency.

With our newfound understanding of the risks associated with hormone depletion, many doctors prescribe hormone-replacement therapy, involving high doses of estrogen and sometimes progesterone. Many women are concerned about conventional estrogen-replacement therapy because some studies show a greater risk of breast cancer in women who use these hormones—primarily when there is a family history of breast cancer. The question of whether or not to take these synthetic hormones is a dilemma.

Knowing your blood type may help you to resolve the conflict and decide which approach is best for your own personal needs.

If you are Type O or Type B and entering menopause, begin to exercise in a manner recommended for your blood type, and in a way appropriate to your current fitness and lifestyle. Eat a high-protein diet. Conventional estrogen replacement generally works reasonably well for Type O and Type B women, unless you have high-risk factors for breast cancer.

If you are Type A or Type AB, you should avoid using conventional estrogen replacement, because of your unusually high susceptibility to breast cancer (see chapter 10). Instead, use the newly available phytoestrogens, which are estrogen- and progesterone-like preparations derived from plants, principally soybeans, alfalfa, and yams. Many of these preparations are available as a cream that can be applied to the skin several times a day. Plant phytoestrogens are typically high in the estrogen fraction called estriol, whereas chemical estrogens are based on estradiol. The medical literature conclusively shows that supplementation with estriol inhibits the occurrence of breast cancer.

Phytoestrogens lack the potency of the chemical estrogens, but they are definitely effective against many of the troubling symptoms of menopause, including hot flashes and vaginal dryness. Because they are only weak estrogens, they will not suppress any estrogen production by the body, unlike the chemical estrogen. For the woman who is not taking any estrogen supplementation because of a family history of breast cancer, phytoestrogens are a godsend. Talk to your gynecologist about using these preparations. If you have no special risk factors for breast cancer, the stronger chemical estrogen is more effective for reducing heart disease and osteoporosis, in addition to the symptoms of menopause.

It is interesting that in Japan, where the typical diet is high in phytoestrogens, there is no concise Japanese word for menopause. Undoubtedly the widespread use of soy products, which contain the phytoestrogens genestein and diaziden, serves to modulate the severe symptoms of menopause.

CASE HISTORY: MENSTRUAL PROBLEMS
Patty, 45: Type O

Patty was a forty-five-year-old African-American woman with a variety of problems, including arthritis, high blood pressure, and severe premenstrual syndrome with heavy bleeding. I first met Patty in December 1994, when she came to my office accompanied by her husband. At the time, she was being treated by one drug or another for her ailments. I learned that Patty had been consuming a basically vegetarian diet, so it was no surprise that she was also anemic. I recommended that she begin exercising, adopt the Type O high-protein diet, and prescribed a course of botanical medicines.

Within two months, Patty made an astounding turnabout. Arthritis: cured. Hypertension: under control. PMS: last two periods, all symptoms gone. Menstrual flow: normal.

I wish it were possible to supply you with a more detailed and complete list of diseases. Perhaps then we could more fully estimate their link to blood type.

The cause and effect of disease often crosses all boundaries. Cancer, for instance, seems to snatch at both the young and old thoughtlessly and without regard to circumstance or exposure.

It is clear, however, that there are many diseases that show a strong propensity for a specific blood type. I hope the evidence I've offered in this discussion of blood type and disease has proven the relationship.

If nothing else, knowing your chances, assessing your risk factors, and understanding the situation gives you another way to take positive action against forces that may often leave you feeling without control.

Now let's look at cancer. Cancer is such a major cause of death and disease—and has such a clear-cut blood type connection—that I'm devoting an entire chapter to its discussion.

TEN

Blood Type
and Cancer:

The Fight to Heal

I EXPERIENCE A PARTICULAR SURGE OF PASSION WHENEVER I examine the healing connection between blood type and cancer. My mother died of breast cancer ten years ago, after an agonizing experience.

My mother was a wonderful woman, whose simple Spanish values guarded us all against any pretense or pomp.

Mom was an anomaly in our family—a Type A who ate what she chose to eat. She had the notorious Catalan strong will. In her house (my parents were divorced), she served a basic Mediterranean diet of meats and salads and some processed foods. In spite of my father's blood type work, there wasn't a soy bean or a legume in sight when we stayed with Mother.

Anyone who has seen a family member or friend engage in a valiant but ultimately fruitless struggle against cancer knows that there is nothing quite so heartbreaking. Watching my mother as she went from mastectomy to chemotherapy to brief remission to recurrence, I could almost visualize the armies of invisible invaders, stealing their way into her healthy cells and gaining a strong foothold before sweeping through her immune system, like barbarians waging a surprise attack. In the end, nothing could be done to stop them. They won.

In the years since my mother's death, I have found myself returning again and again to the mysteries of cancer. I have often wondered whether my mother might have been spared had she adhered to a Type A Diet, or whether she was somehow genetically preselected to fight and lose this battle. I have dedicated myself to finding those answers on her behalf. You might say I have a Catalan-style vendetta against breast cancer, above all other cancers.

Does cancer find an inherently more fertile ground to grow and develop in the body of one blood type than in another? The answer is a definite yes.

There is undeniable evidence that persons with Type A or Type AB blood have an overall higher rate of cancer and poorer odds of survival than Type O and Type B. Actually, as early as the 1940s, the American Medical Association stated that Type AB had the greatest rate of cancer of all the blood types, but the news didn't make headlines, probably because Type ABs constitute such a low percentage of the population. Statistically, their high numbers didn't cause the same kind of alarm as the information about the more common Type A. But from a personal standpoint, that's surely of little comfort to the individuals with Type AB blood. Researchers may treat cancer like a numbers game; I prefer to treat it as a personal crisis in the life of a single individual.

Type O and Type B show much lower incidences of cancer, but we don't yet have enough information to say exactly why that is. There are important clues, however, in the antigen and antibody activity of the different blood types that we can explore.

Having said that, the blood type–cancer connection is highly complex and in many ways mysterious. Be clear that being Type AB or Type A doesn't mean it's certain or even likely that you personally are going to get cancer, any more than being Type O or Type B means you'll absolutely be spared. There are many causes of cancer, and we are still haunted by the mystery of why some people with no seeming risk factors, contract the disease.

Increasingly, blood type has emerged as a vital factor, but it is only one piece of the puzzle. There are many causes of cancer—chemical carcinogens, radiation, and other genetic factors, to name a few. These factors are largely independent of blood type, and as such would not produce enough of a difference in the population to be able to be predicted by blood type alone. For example, cigarette smoking could easily mask or weaken a blood type association because it is a powerful enough carcinogen to cause cancer all by itself—regardless of your inherent susceptibility or lack of it.

There is an enormous amount of scientific research on the molecular relationship between blood type and cancer. But the research has practically ignored the question of whether a person with one blood type or another has a better chance of surviving particular cancers.

Who lives and who dies? Who survives and who doesn't? This, in my opinion, is the great missing link in the research on cancer and blood type. The real blood type–cancer connection resides in the rates of resolution rather than in the rates of occurrence among the different blood types. And that connection may be the glue of lectins.

The Cancer-Lectin Connection

SHAKESPEARE once wrote, "There is some soul of goodness in things evil." In some instances, like chemotherapy treatments to fight cancer, it is expedient and even beneficial to use a poison. In relationship to cancer, lectins serve two purposes: They can be used to agglutinate cancerous cells, thus acting as a catalyst for the immune system—a wake-up call to get busy and protect the good cells.

How does this happen? Under normal circumstances, the production of surface sugars by a cell is highly specific and controlled. Not in a cancer cell. Because the genetic material is scrambled, cancer cells lose control over the production of their

The Lectin-Cancer Connection

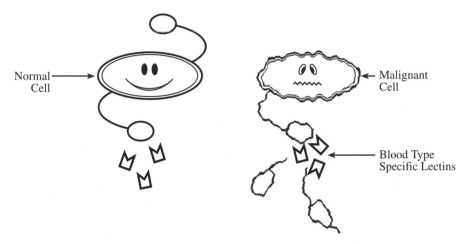

Normal Cell

Malignant Cell

Blood Type Specific Lectins

Why lectins agglutinate cancer cells. The cells depicted on the left side of the drawing represent non-malignant cells. Because the production of surface sugars is controlled by intact genetic material, normal cell walls have surface sugars arranged in an orderly pattern. But malignant cells have many more surface sugars because their genetic material is flawed, resulting in the malignant cell producing uncontrolled amounts of these sugars. If a blood type–specific food lectin is added to a suspension of normal and malignant cells, it will interact more aggressively with the "fuzzier" malignant cells than with the "smoother" normal cells.

surface sugars, and usually manufacture them in greater amounts than a normal cell would. Cancer cells are more liable than normal cells to tangle up if they come in contact with the appropriate lectin.

Malignant cancerous cells are as much as 100 times more sensitive to the agglutinating effects of lectins than normal cells. If two slides are prepared, one containing normal cells and the other malignant, an equal dose of the appropriate lectin will convert the slide with malignant cells into a huge entangled clump, whereas the slide of normal cells will show little, if any, change.

When malignant cells become agglutinated into huge tangles of hundreds, thousands, or millions of cancer cells, the immune system becomes reactivated. Now the antibodies can target the clumps of cancer cells, identifying them for destruction. This search-and-destroy mission is usually carried out by powerful scavenger cells found in the liver.

If you were to go into a medical database and key in lectins and cancer, the printer would be working overtime for days. Lectins are extensively used to study the molecular biology of cancer because they make excellent probes, helping to identify unique antigens, called markers, on the surface of the cancer cells. Beyond this, their use is limited, which is a shame because they are so ubiquitous in common foods. By identifying the blood type of a person with a particular cancer, and using the appropriate lectins derived from the Blood Type Diet, a powerful new tool can be utilized by any cancer patient to improve their odds of survival.

Enter the Blood Type

AN ENORMOUS amount of cell division occurs in the course of one's lifetime. Given these odds, it is amazing that more cancer doesn't occur. This is probably because the immune system has a special ability to detect and eliminate the vast majority of mutations that take place on a day-to-day basis. Cancer probably results from a breakdown in this surveillance, the successful cancer cell tricking the immune system into impotency by mimicking normal cells. As we have already seen, the blood types possess unique powers of surveillance, depending on the shape and form of the intruder.

This gives you a rough idea of how blood types, agglutinating lectins, and cancer interact together. The obvious next question is: What does it mean? And if you are personally worried about cancer, What does this mean for you?

I'll level with you: To date, the only cancer for which we have substantial information about the blood type connection is breast cancer. I will talk about it in fairly substantial detail. The other cancers are less well defined regarding blood types, but we do have limited information that I will share. We also know that there are many food-related links that undoubtedly apply to all, or most, cancers, and we'll study these carefully in light of what we know about nutrition and blood types. There are also some innovative naturopathic therapies that are gaining wider favor and are held in high regard.

The research goes on, but it is an agonizingly slow process. Even now, as I write this, I am beginning the eighth year of a ten-year trial on reproductive cancers, using the Blood Type Diets. My results are encouraging. So far, the women in my trial have double the survival rate published by the American Cancer Society. By the time I release the results in another two years, I expect to make it scientifically demonstrable that the Blood Type Diet plays a role in cancer remission.

The work goes on. The more we learn, the more we live. Let me tell you what I've discovered—about the cancers themselves, and then about what steps you can take.

Breast Cancer

A number of years ago, while taking histories on new patients, I began to notice that many women who had suffered from breast cancer at some time in their distant pasts and had fully recovered were Type Os or Type Bs. Their rate of recovery was especially impressive since most of them told me that their treatment had not been very aggressive—usually no more than surgical excision, only rarely including radiation or chemotherapy.

How could this be? The statistics on breast cancer show that, even with the most aggressive treatment, only 19 to 25 percent of the women survive five to ten years after the diagnosis. Yet these women had survived for a much longer time with only minimal therapy. Was it possible that being Type O or Type B helped to protect them against the spread of the disease or a recurrence?

Over the years, I also began to notice a distinct tendency in Type A women with breast cancer—and also in Type AB women, although I haven't seen many with that rare blood type—to suffer from a more aggressive malignancy and a lower survival rate, even when biopsies taken from the lymph nodes showed that they were free of cancer. Through my own clinical experiences and study of scientific literature, I concluded that there is a major connection between surviving breast cancer and your blood type.

In 1991, a study appeared in the *Lancet*, an English medical journal, that may have provided part of the answer. Researchers reported that it appeared possible to predict whether or not a breast cancer would spread to the lymph nodes by virtue of its characteristics when treated with a stain containing a lectin from the edible snail *Helix pomatia*. They reported a strong association between the uptake of the snail lectin and the subsequent development of metastasis to the lymph nodes. In other words, antigens on the surface of the primary breast cancer cells were changing, and this change was allowing the cancer to spread into the lymph nodes. Now, here comes the punch line: the lectin of *Helix pomatia* is highly specific—to Blood Type A.

The researchers studying breast cancer discovered that as the cancer cells changed, they made themselves more A-like. This allowed them to bypass all of the body's defenses and rage unimpeded into the defenseless lymph.

Did my Type O patients survive because they were Type O? Did my Type B patients survive because they were Type B? It certainly looked that way.

And there is a confirmation in our scientific understanding of cancer. Many tumor cells have unique antigens, or markers, on their surfaces. For instance, breast cancer patients often show high levels of Cancer Antigen 15-3 (CA15-3), a marker for breast cancer, ovarian cancer patients often have high levels of Cancer Antigen 125 (CA125); while prostate cancer patients can have an elevated Prostate Specific Antigen (PSA); and so on. These antigens are often used to track the progress of the disease and effectiveness of treatment, and are called tumor markers. Many tumor markers possess blood type activity. Sometimes the tumor markers are incomplete or corrupted blood type antigens, which in a normal cell would have gone on to form a part of the person's blood type system.

Not surprisingly, many of these tumor markers have A-like qualities, which allow them easy access to the Type A and Type

AB systems. There they are welcomed as self—the ultimate molecular Trojan horse. Obviously, the A-like intruders would be more easily detected and eliminated if they were to slip into a Type O or Type B system.

Breast cancer markers are overwhelmingly A-like. That's the answer to my question about the differing rates of recurrence on the part of my patients. Although my Type O and Type B patients had developed breast cancer, their anti-A antigens were better able to fight it off, rounding up the early cancer cells and destroying them. On the other hand, my Type A and Type AB patients couldn't fight as well because they couldn't see their opponents. Everywhere they turned, the cells looked just like them—and they were unable to detect the mutated cancer cells beneath their clever masks.

CASE HISTORY: PREVENTING BREAST CANCER
Anne, 47: Type A

Four years ago Anne came to the office for a general wellness visit, without any real physical complaints. But while I was doing her medical history, I learned that Anne's family had a high incidence of breast cancer on both her mother's and father's sides—and the mortality rate among those who had the disease was very high.

Anne knew about her genetic risk factors, but she was surprised to learn that her Type A blood presented an additional risk factor. "I don't suppose it makes any difference, though," she said. "Either I'm going to get breast cancer or I'm not. There's nothing I can really do about it."

I advised Anne that there were several measures she could take. First, because of her family history, she needed to be hypervigilant about suspicious breast lumps, perform frequent breast self-examinations, and make sure to get routine mammograms.

"When was your last mammogram?" I asked. Anne sheepishly told me that her last mammogram had been seven years before. It

turned out that Anne was strongly disinclined to avail herself of
any conventional medical techniques. She had educated herself
about herbs and vitamins, and often used them to treat herself effectively. But when it came to more intrusive medical treatments,
she shied away. However, she did promise to schedule a mammogram.

Anne's mammogram was clean, and she began a concentrated
program of cancer avoidance. The Type A Diet was an easy tran-
sition for Anne because she already ate a primarily vegetarian diet.
I fine-tuned the diet with anti-cancer foods—especially increasing the amount of soy, and adding specific naturopathic herbs.
Anne began to study yoga. She told me that for the first time in
her adult life, she wasn't constantly worrying about cancer.

A year later, Anne had a second mammogram. This time a
suspicious mark was detected in her left breast. A biopsy showed
it to be a precancerous condition known as neoplasia. Essentially,
neoplasia is the presence of mutated cells. It's not cancer, but it
can become cancer if the cells continue to deteriorate and multiply. During the biopsy, Anne's doctor completely removed the
pre-cancerous mark.

Three years later, there have been no new growths detected,
although we are watching Anne very carefully. She continues to
follow the Type A Diet religiously, and says she has never felt
healthier.

Of all the functions a physician can perform, none is more elegant and valuable than successful prediction and intervention. I
was glad Anne came to me when she did, and that she took all the
right steps.

The Antigen Vaccine

BREAST CANCER continues to be a baffling and too often deadly.
But there are some signs that blood type may represent a key to
the cure.

Dr. George Springer, a research scientist with the Bligh Cancer Center at the University of Chicago School of Medicine, has been investigating the effects of a vaccine whose basis is a molecule called the T antigen. Since the 1950s, Springer has been one of the most important investigators in the role of blood type to disease. His contributions to the field are phenomenal. His work on the T antigen has been most promising.

The T antigen is a common tumor marker found in many cancers, especially breast cancer. Healthy, cancer-free people carry antibodies against the T antigen, so it is never seen in them.

Springer believes that a vaccine composed of the T antigen and the tumor marker CA15-3 can help jolt and then reawaken the suppressed immune systems of cancer patients, helping them attack and destroy the cancerous cells. For the past twenty years, Springer and his colleagues have been using a vaccine derived from the T antigen as a long-term treatment against the recurrence of advanced breast cancer. Although the study group is small—less than twenty-five women—the results are impressive. All of the eleven breast cancer patients with severely advanced disease (Stage III and Stage IV), survived for longer than five years—remarkable in what is considered end-stage cancer; while six of them (three Stage III and three Stage IV) survived from ten to eighteen years. These results are nothing short of miraculous.

Springer's continued work on blood type systems and cancer convinces me that the natural evolution of our understanding of blood types will eventually provide not just information on risk factors, but also a cure for every manifestation of the disease.

Other Forms of Cancer

THE PATHOLOGY of this disease—wild marauders out for a night on the town—is fundamentally the same in all cancers. Yet there are variations related both to cause and to blood type. The A-like or B-like tumor markers exert remarkable control over the way the body's immune system reacts to the cancer's invasion and growth.

Again, almost all cancers show a preference for Type A and

Type AB, although there are occasional forms that are B-like—such as female reproductive and bladder cancers. Type Os seem to be far more resistant to developing almost any cancer. Intolerant and hostile, I believe that Type Os more simple fucose sugars dispose them to tossing off the A-like—or in some cases, B-like—cancer cells, and developing anti-A or anti-B antibodies.

Again, we unfortunately know little about the full implications of the blood type link in cancers other than breast cancer. However, it most likely follows a similar course. Let's examine some of the most common forms of cancer:

BRAIN TUMORS. Most cancers of the brain and nervous system, such as glioma multiforma and astrocytoma, show a preference for Type A and Type AB. Their tumor markers are A-like.

FEMALE REPRODUCTIVE CANCERS. Cancers of the female reproductive system (uterine, cervical, ovarian, and labial) show a preference for Type A and Type AB women. However, there is also a numerically high number of Type B women who suffer from these cancers. This implies that there are different tumor markers created, depending upon the circumstances. Ovarian cysts and uterine fibroids, which are usually benign but may be a sign of susceptibility to cancer, generate copious amounts of Type A and Type B antigens.

As I mentioned earlier, I am currently in the eighth year of a ten-year clinical trial of women with reproductive cancer. Most of my patients are Type A, and a few are Type B. Only occasionally do I treat a Type AB woman, probably because there aren't very many of them.

COLON CANCER. Blood type is not the strongest determinant for the various forms of colon cancer. The real risk factors for the conditions that lead to colon cancer are related to diet, lifestyle, and temperament. Ulcerative colitis, Crohn's disease, and irritable bowel syndrome left unmitigated eventually leave the system depleted and open to cancer. A high-fat diet, combined with smoking and alcohol consumption, create the ideal environment for digestive cancers. The risk is greater if you have a family history of colon cancer.

MOUTH AND UPPER DIGESTIVE CANCERS. Cancers of the lip, tongue, gums, and cheek; tumors of the salivary gland; and esophageal cancer are all strongly linked to Type A and Type AB. Most of these cancers are self-generated, in that the risks can be minimized if you abstain from tobacco, moderate your alcohol consumption, and watch your diet.

STOMACH AND ESOPHAGEAL CANCER. Stomach cancer is attracted to low levels of stomach acid, a Type A and Type AB trait. In well over 63,000 cases of stomach cancer studied, Type A and Type AB were predominant.

Stomach cancer is epidemic in China, Japan, and Korea because the typical diet is rich in smoked, pickled, and fermented foods. These Asian dietary staples seem to counter any of the good that soybeans might do, perhaps because they are packed with carcinogenic nitrates. Asian Type Bs, who have higher levels of stomach acid, aren't as prone to stomach cancer, even if they eat some of the same foods.

PANCREATIC, LIVER, GALLBLADDER, AND BILE DUCT CANCERS. These cancers are rare in Type Os, with their hardy digestive systems. Type A and Type AB are at most risk, with Type Bs having some susceptibility—especially if they consume many "harsh" foods such as nuts and seeds.

Several of the earlier therapies for these cancers included large portions of fresh liver from sheep, horse, and buffalo. They seemed to help, but no one knew why. It was later discovered that the livers contained lectins that slowed the growth and spread of pancreatic, liver, gallbladder, and bile duct cancers.

CASE HISTORY: LIVER CANCER
Cathy, 49: Type A

Cathy first sought medical attention in the late 1980s for a suspicious growth in her abdomen, which turned out to be an aggressive form of liver cancer. She was treated at Harvard's Deaconess Hospital in Boston, Massachusetts, and eventually received a liver transplant. She was referred to me in 1990.

In the subsequent two years, most of my focus was on using naturopathic techniques to replace the immunosuppressing anti-rejection drugs needed to help her keep her transplanted liver. Cathy's condition improved to the point where she was able to stop her drug therapy.

However, in 1992, Cathy noticed some shortness of breath, and at her checkup at Harvard, doctors noticed suspicious lesions on her chest X ray. These turned out to be cancer.

Cathy and her physicians were on the horns of a dilemma. Her lungs were so heavily laced with cancer, surgery was out of the question ("It would be like picking cherries," said her surgeon), and her liver transplant ruled out chemotherapy.

We went to work, using the basic Type A–lectin cancer diet and other immune-enhancing botanicals. I also recommended a preparation made from shark cartilage for Cathy to take orally and use as an enema.

In an amazing series of correspondences, Cathy's surgical team at Harvard kept me up to date on her progress. In a letter dated September 3, 1992, I was informed that the lesions in Cathy's lung had shrunk and looked more like scar tissue. Subsequent letters confirmed these findings. By 1993, even the scar tissue had begun to disappear.

Cathy was stunned and overjoyed. "When they told me that the cancer seemed to be going into remission, I felt as if I had won the lottery," she said happily. Cathy went on to live three symptom-free years, Unfortunately, her cancer returned at that point, and she later died.

The case is especially interesting for two reasons: First,

throughout this time Cathy received no treatment other than naturopathic. Second, her team at Harvard was open-minded and supportive of her using a naturopathic doctor. Perhaps what we have seen here is a tiny glimpse of the future: all medical systems working together for the betterment of the patient.

By the way, the total cost of Cathy's naturopathic therapy was less than $1,500, as opposed to the tens of thousands she might have spent on conventional treatment.

Lymphomas, Leukemias, and Hodgkin's Disease. This is a form of cancer to which Type Os are predisposed— maybe. Although these cancers of the blood and lymph preferentially afflict Type Os, they may not be true cancers at all, but rather viral infections that have run amok. This would make some sense in light of what we know about Type Os; they're actually pretty good at fighting most cancers, but the Type O antigen is not well designed for fighting viruses.

Lung Cancer. Lung cancer is truly nonspecific. It is one of the few cancers which has no particular blood type connection. Lung cancer is most commonly caused by cigarette smoking.

Yes, lung cancer is caused by many other things as well. There are people who have never smoked who will die of lung cancer as you are reading this sentence. But we all know that smoking is the overwhelming cause of lung cancer. Tobacco is such a powerful carcinogen in its own right that it bypasses anything so obvious, so ordered as predilection.

Prostate Cancer. There appears to be a higher level of prostate cancer in secretors (see Appendix E). My own experience has been that a greater number of Type A and Type AB men suffer from prostate cancer than do Type O or Type B men. A Type A or Type AB secretor is at the highest risk.

Skin and Bone Cancers. Skin cancers are unique in that there is a greater number of Type Os who suffer from them. Per-

haps the lighter skins of northern Europeans—who are predomi-
nantly Type Os—are reacting to the increasing levels of ultraviolet radiation caused by environmental pollution.

Malignant melanoma is the deadliest form of skin cancer.
Type A and Type AB are at greatest risk for this condition, although Type O and Type B are not immune.

Bone cancers seem to show a consistent preference for Type
B, although there is some risk for Type A and Type AB.

URINARY TRACT CANCER. Bladder cancer in both men and
women occurs most often in Type A and Type B. Type ABs, who
have the double whammy of both A and B characteristics, are
probably at the greatest risk of all.

Far more than Type As, Type Bs who suffer from recurrent
bladder and kidney infection should be especially careful with
the management of this problem, as it inevitably leads to more
serious disease.

One puzzling connection that is yet to be unraveled: wheat
germ agglutinin, the lectin that can act favorably against both lobular and intraductal breast cancers, paradoxically accelerates the
growth of bladder cancer cells.

Fighting Back

CANCER ALWAYS seems to present a discouraging picture. I imagine
that if you are Type A or Type AB, you may be thinking grim
thoughts. Remember, though, that susceptibility is a single factor
among many. I believe that knowing your predilection for cancer,
and understanding the workings of your specific blood type, gives
you more opportunity than you would otherwise have to fight
back. The following strategies can give you a way to make a difference for yourself, especially if you are Type A or Type AB. In
particular, many of the foods suggested are tailored for these
blood types. Current research has focused primarily on the A-like

markers for breast cancer, and little investigation has been conducted regarding the B-like cancers. Unfortunately, this means that while the cancer-fighting foods suggested here may be very effective for Type As and Type ABs, they won't necessarily help Type Bs or Type Os. In fact, most of these foods (peanuts, lentils, and wheat germ) cause other problems for these two blood types.

The clinical trials I am currently conducting, along with the work of other scientists and researchers, will one day give us a deeper understanding of the cancer-diet connection for all the blood types. In the meantime, Type Bs and Type Os can reduce the chance of the cell mutations that can lead to cancer by adhering to your blood type diet. If you already have a cancerous condition, take special note of the other therapies in this section, especially the pneumovax vaccine. Further research will offer a more complete picture.

1. You Live as You Eat
People with Type A blood have digestive tracts that find it difficult to break down animal fats and proteins. Type As and Type ABs should adhere to a diet high in fiber and low in animal products.

There are specific foods that must be given extra consideration as cancer preventives.

SOYBEANS . . . AGAIN
Three to 11 percent of every cake of tofu is composed of soybean agglutinins. Soybean agglutinins are able to selectively identify early mutated cells producing the Type A antigen and sweep them from the system —while leaving normal Type A cells alone. Although soy foods are a rich source, only a minute amount is needed for agglutination.

The soybean agglutinin especially discriminates when it comes to breast cancer cells; it is so specific that it's been used to remove cancerous cells from harvested bone marrow. In experimental work with breast cancer patients, their bone marrow was removed. They were then bombarded with high levels of chemotherapy and radiation. These oncology tools would normally destroy the bone marrow. Instead, the harvested marrow—cleansed by the soybean lectin— was then reintroduced into the patient. These treatments have shown some very good results. The soybean lectin also contains the estrogen-related compounds genestein and diaziden. These compounds not only help to balance the effect of a woman's estrogen levels, but also contain other properties which can help reduce the blood supply to tumor cells.

Soybeans in all forms are beneficial to Type As and Type ABs as a general cancer preventative. The vegetable proteins in soy are easier for these blood types to utilize, and so it is strongly suggested that these blood types reexamine any aversion they may have to tofu and tofu products. Think of tofu not only as a food, but as a powerful medicine. Although Type Bs can eat soy foods, it is not certain whether they have the same action in the Type B bloodstream.

Japanese women have such a low incidence of breast cancer because the use of tofu and other soy products is still high in the overall Japanese diet. As the diet becomes more Westernized, it is possible that we will see a proportionate rise in certain forms of cancer. One study of Japanese immigrant women living in San Francisco showed that they had twice the rate of breast cancer as their cousins living in Japan—no doubt due to a change in dietary habits.

Peanuts

The peanut agglutinin has also been found to contain a specific lectin sensitive to breast cancer cells, particularly the medullary form. The peanut lectin shows activity to a lesser degree against all other forms, including intraductal, lobular, and scirrhous breast cancers. This connection is probably true of other A-like cancers.

Eat fresh peanuts with the skins still on them; the skins, not the shells. Peanut butter is probably not a good source of the lectin, as the majority of brands are just too processed and homogenized.

LENTILS
The *Lens culinaris* lectin found in common domestic brown or green lentils shows a strong specific attraction for lobular, medullary, intraductal, and stromal forms of breast cancer, and is likely to affect other A-like cancers.

LIMA BEANS
Lima bean lectin is one of the most potent agglutinants of all Type A cells, cancerous or not. When you're healthy, lima beans will hurt you—so they shouldn't be part of a prevention strategy. However, if you are suffering from an A-like cancer, eat the lima beans. The lectin will agglutinate untold numbers of cancer cells. It will also destroy some perfectly innocent and upstanding Type A cells, but the exchange is worth it.

WHEAT GERM
Wheat germ agglutinin shows a great affinity for Type A cancers. The wheat germ agglutinin is concentrated in the seed coating, the outer husk that is usually discarded. Unprocessed wheat bran will provide the most significant quantity of the lectin, although you can also use commercial wheat germ preparations.

SNAILS
If you're Type A or Type AB, order escargots the next time you dine at a fancy French restaurant. Consider it medicine packaged in a glamorous, delicious form.

The edible snail, *Helix pomatia*, is a powerful breast cancer agglutinin capable of determining whether the cancerous cells will metastasize to the lymph nodes.

Unless the thought of eating snails disgusts you (and really, they're quite delicious), what harm can it do?

2. Other Strategies
TAKE CARE OF YOUR LIVER AND COLON
Women should be aware that the liver and colon are two major sites where estrogens can be degraded—if their functions are disturbed,

the levels of estrogen throughout the body can rise. Elevated estrogen activity can stimulate the growth of cancerous cells.

Adopt a high-fiber diet to increase the levels of butyrate in the colon wall cells. Butyrates, as you may recall, promote the normalization of tissue.

The grain amaranth also contains a lectin that has a specific affinity to colon cancer cells and will destroy them.

T HE   P NEUMOVAX   V ACCINE

Pneumovax (pneumococcus vaccine) elevates anti–Type A antibodies. Type Os and Type Bs produced higher levels of anti-A antibodies when given this vaccine, making them even better able to fight A-like cancers. This is the first promising treatment for Type Bs and Type Os who have cancer. In effect, it allows you to strengthen your defenses against A-like cancerous mutations, making you even better prepared to fight specific cancers such as breast, stomach, liver, and pancreatic cancers.

Type As obviously will not produce anti-A antibodies, but the Pneumovax may give a boost to their immune systems, helping them to recognize cancerous cells normally incognito. Since most cancers have A-like tendencies, the Pneumovax may, by elevating anti–Type A antibodies, mobilize the immune systems of all the blood types.

Several further positives that the pneumococcus vaccine offers: it is safe; it is inexpensive; it prevents some forms of pneumonia; and most important, it generates isohemaglutinins.

Isohemaglutinins are much more powerful antibodies than those the body manufactures against a virus or a bacteria. Isohemaglutinins are "Terminators." They agglutinate and kill their prey by themselves, requiring no assistance from the other normal killer cells of the immune system. Isohemaglutinins float through the bloodstream like innocent snowflakes, but when they attach to cells they change form to become three-dimensional, crablike antibodies. They are so prominent that they can be detected by a microscope.

Blood Type O and Type B can really rev up their anti-A antibodies with a Pneumovax every eight to ten years. Blood Type A and Type AB should revaccinate more often, every five years.

ANTIOXIDANTS

There has been so much conflicting information about antioxidants, their purported benefits or lack of them, that it's difficult to recommend the best combinations.

Vitamin antioxidants have been studied for breast cancer, and have been shown to be not very effective in preventing the disease. Vitamin E and beta-carotenes don't deposit in high enough concentrations in breast tissue to effect positive change.

The plant-based antioxidants do seem to make some difference, but must be combined with supplemental sources of vitamin C to synergize for greatest effect. Yellow onions contain very high levels of quercetin, an especially potent antioxidant. It has none of the estrogenizing activity of vitamin E, and is hundreds of times stronger than vitamin antioxidants. Quercitin is available as a supplement in many health food stores.

Women with a risk factor for breast cancer who are considering or are on estrogen-replacement therapy, should use phytoestrogens derived from natural products instead of synthetic estrogens. Plant-based estrogens contain high levels of estriol, a weaker form of the estrogen hormone than estradiol, which is manufactured synthetically. Estriol seems to lower your chances of developing breast cancer. The synthetics increase the risk.

Tamoxifen, an estrogen-blocking drug prescribed to breast cancer patients with estrogen-sensitive breast tumors, is itself a weaker form of estrogen. Genestein is an estrogen-related compound found in the soybean lectin. This phytoestrogen inhibits angiogenesis, interfering with the production of new blood vessels needed to feed the growth of cancerous tumors.

GENERAL PALLIATIVES

Exercise frequently. Get adequate rest. Avoid known pollutants and pesticides. Eat your fruits and vegetables. Type As and Type ABs, eat plenty of tofu. Don't use antibiotics indiscriminately. If you get sick, allow your immune system to fight off the illness. You'll be much healthier if you do, rather than relying on flu shots or antibiotics. They suppress your immune system's natural responses, which can be very powerful if given the chance.

CASE HISTORY: ADVANCED BREAST CANCER
Jane, 50: Type AB

I first saw Jane in my office in April 1993. She had already had a mastectomy and several rounds of chemotherapy for an infiltrating ductal breast cancer that extensively seeded into the lymph nodes. At the time of her initial diagnosis, Jane had two separate tumors on her left breast—one 4 cm and the other 1.5 cm. No one was holding out any great hope for her long-term survival.

I put Jane on the modified cancer diet for Type AB, with an emphasis on soy (high in A lectins), had her Pneumovaxed, and put her on the botanical protocol I use for Type As with breast cancer. Her tumor marker, the CA15-3, which was 166 when she came in (normal is less than 10) dropped almost immediately to 87 in June, and to 34 in August. I recommended that she go see George Springer in Chicago to see if she could get into his vaccine study, which she did.

To this day all signs, including bone scans, look promising, although as Jane is a Type AB, I would be wary to pronounce her cured at this point. Only time will tell.

Cancer prevention and natural immune-system enhancement offer the brightest hope for the future. Genetic research is bringing us ever closer to being able to understand—perhaps someday even control—the cellular workings of this astounding machine that we call our bodies.

Scientists at the National Institute of Allergy and Infectious Diseases in Bethesda, Maryland, announced on May 9, 1996, that they had found a protein used to allow the AIDS virus entry into the immune system. This discovery could be used to someday test new drugs and vaccines targeted at the AIDS virus and many cancers. This exciting breakthrough also helps to explain why some people infected with the AIDS virus remain healthy and disease free for years, while others quickly succumb to its ravages. Wouldn't it be remarkable if the tragic scourge of AIDS led us to a cure for cancer?

Cancer has long been among the most dreaded diseases of mankind. We seem powerless to protect ourselves and those we love from its clinging and relentless grip. Blood type analysis allows us a deeper understanding of our susceptibilities. By consciously examining our exposures to both environmental and dietary carcinogens, and changing some of our lifestyle and food choices, we can minimize the effects of cell damage.

Blood type analysis also provides a way to enhance the ability of the immune system to search out and destroy cancerous and mutated cells while they are few in number. Cancer patients can use their knowledge of blood type to fully develop the capabilities of their immune systems to fight the disease. They can also gain a greater understanding of the mechanisms involved in the growth and spread of cancer.

The treatments for cancer are still far from perfect, although many people have been saved by the latest advances in therapy and scientific medical knowledge. For those of you with cancer, and for those of you who have a family history of cancer, the advice is clear: Change your diet, change your attitudes, and start using antioxidant supplements. If you follow these suggestions you will be able to gain more control and a greater peace of mind. We all dread this horrible disease, but we can take positive action against it.

A Wrinkle
of Earth

*T*HE HUMAN JOURNEY BEGAN AS ONE PEOPLE OF ONE blood—Type O, the blood of our first ancestors. It is an ineffable mystery as to precisely when the first Type A appeared, or the mother and father of Type B, or even when the very recent Type AB was first created. We just don't know; we can only see the broad brushstrokes of history, not its fine details.

But we are always learning. Today, the Human Genome Project employs the most sophisticated technologies in its quest to map the entire genetic structure of the human body—to name, gene by gene, chromosome by chromosome, the purpose of each living cell in the grand scheme of some Master Builder. Thus far, many breakthroughs have come in our understanding of the vast cellular networks of which we are composed—among them, the discovery of a gene for breast cancer. In late May of 1996 the Project announced that they had just isolated and identified the gene responsible for arthritis. Soon, we will be able to control our genetic fates as never before.

Or will we?

Evolution can be defined as an unfolding over time. In the

waning days of the twentieth century, what is there left for us to unfold? The Hubble Telescope peers into the farthest reaches of a seemingly endless universe aswirl in uncharted galaxies; scientists then announce that 400 or 500 billion more galaxies exist than they had previously calculated. They also announce that the observable universe extends at least 15 billion light-years—in every direction.

The World Wide Web beckons. Communications have become almost instantaneous. There has been an explosion of knowledge in all fields, with much more to come. We are a sophisticated, increasingly urbane people. We are at our genetic peak!

Well, so were the Neanderthals once. And for many thousands of years, Cro-Magnon dominated this planet. When the barbarian hordes came rampaging through Europe in wave after wave of invasion, it must have seemed to those invaded that it would never end. But our lives and our memories are short. We are without substance in the flame of endless time, gossamer shredding in the wind. The revolution is not over. It is still taking place.

Evolution is very subtle. Our genetic makeups and those of our children, and those of our children's children, continue to alter in infinitesimal and unknown ways of which we are completely unaware. Some may believe that the evolution revolution is over. I am convinced that it is an ongoing, kinetic process.

The Revolution Continues

WHERE DOES the power of life come from? What propels us and compels us to survive?

Our blood. Our life force.

There have been recent outbreaks of rare viruses and infectious diseases as we have pushed into the remaining untouched jungles of this planet. These diseases defy medical intervention. Will our bodies produce answers to the challenges posed by the unknown?

This is what we face:

- Increasing ultraviolet radiation caused by the depletion of the ozone layer . . .
- The increased pollution of our air and water . . .
- Increasing food contamination . . .
- Overpopulation and famine . . .
- Infectious diseases beyond our power to control . . .
- Unknown plagues emerging from all of the above. . . .

We will survive. We have always survived. What form that survival will take, and what the world and its stresses will be like for the survivors, we do not know.

Perhaps a new blood type will emerge—call it Type C. This new blood type will be able to create antibodies to fend off every antigen that exists today, and any future permutation of antigens that develops. In an overcrowded, polluted world with few natural resources left, the new Type Cs will come to dominate their societies. The antiquated blood types will begin to die off in an increasingly hostile environment for which they are no longer suited. Finally, Type C will rule.

Or maybe a different scenario will be played out, one in which our scientific knowledge finally allows us to gain dominion over the worst impulses of humanity, and civilization is able to rouse itself from the suicidal impulses that seem to impel it to doom.

Our knowledge is truly vast, and there is every reason to hope that the finest and most altruistic minds and spirits of our age might focus on a way to deal with the realities of our world—violence, war, crime, ignorance, intolerance, hatred, and disease—and thus pull us out of this toxic spiral.

Nothing is complete. This world and our purpose in it is an ever-changing equation of which each of us is momentarily an integral part. The revolution continues with us or without us. Time sees us only as a blink of the eye, and it is this impermanence that makes our lives so precious.

By sharing my father's fascination with and my scientific knowledge of the Blood Type Diets, I hope to make a positive impact on the life of everyone who examines this book.

Like my father before me, I am a practicing naturopathic physician. I have dedicated myself to the pursuit of naturopathic knowledge and research, and this work has been my passion for many years. It began as a gift from my father and became, for me, a gift to my father. This is the Blood Type Solution, the revolutionary breakthrough that will change the way you eat and live.

A Medical
Breakthrough
for the Ages

by Dr. Joseph Pizzorno,
President, Bastyr University

*T*HIS IS AN INCREDIBLY EXCITING TIME FOR NAT-
ural medicine. Finally, modern medical science has developed
the analytical tools and information base to understand the mechanisms of centuries-old healing wisdom. While many theories on
health prevail worldwide, only a small number have been subjected to scientific scrutiny, as few natural healers have either the
technical skills or the emotional inclination to study the research
literature. For natural medicine to become established as an integral part of today's health care systems, it must fulfill the expec-
tations of the modern world for reliability and credibility.

Bastyr University in Seattle, Washington, has shown how to do
this. Founded in 1978, Bastyr's mission has been to bring to the
world the benefits of credible, science-based natural medicine.
Bastyr provides accredited cutting-edge education, insightful research, and effective clinical services in naturopathic medicine.
Its graduates are leaders in their fields.

Dr. Peter D'Adamo, a graduate of our first class of naturopathic physicians in 1982, is an outstanding example of the best
Bastyr has to offer. His exciting pioneering work could change

the practice of medicine for centuries to come. Inspired by his father's preliminary theories about the importance of blood type in predicting a person's biochemistry, Peter worked with students at Bastyr for over a decade, culling over 1,000 papers from the scientific research literature. This exhaustive study of medical and anthropological research, combined with clinical observation and scientific inquiry, matured into a cohesive theory with a credible foundation. The rational guidelines Peter developed will fundamentally enhance people's health and afford a deeper understanding of how an individual's genetic background determines his biochemistry and dictates his susceptibility to disease and environmental factors, including diet. This work will surely provide valuable insights for physicians responsible for the treatment of many of today's most challenging diseases.

I was first exposed to the unique concept of using blood types to better understand an individual's unique dietary and biochemical needs when Peter was a student at Bastyr. One of the courses I taught in the naturopathic medicine program required students to carefully research a topic of interest to them and then present it, in both written and oral form, to the rest of the class. During a particularly memorable class in 1981, Peter stimulated considerable excitement and intense discussion when he presented the unexpected concept his father had intuitively developed—that blood type could be a determining factor in health. As might be expected, many more questions were asked than Peter could answer. The high level of interest and large number of insightful questions appeared to especially engage Peter's own intellectual curiosity, stimulating him to commence his important quest.

Over the next several years, Peter engaged in a considerable amount of study and research. I remember many fascinating conversations with him resulting in my recruiting several of our better graduate students at Bastyr to help him comb the medical and anthropological research journals. As the years progressed, Peter called often to share his excitement as he uncovered the surprising amount of relevant research that had been performed in a wide range of disciplines. But until Peter, no one had put it all together or thought through the implications of what different researchers were discovering.

His studies culminated in his landmark presentation at the 1989 Annual Convention of the American Association of Naturopathic Physicians in Rippling River, Oregon. The audience was extremely excited by the clinical applicability, and a lively discussion followed. Since then many leading clinicians have adopted Peter's blood type–based protocols.

Hippocrates is said to have stated: "Let your medicines be your foods and your foods your medicine." But how to do this? One of the most significant challenges facing the dedicated physician is how to determine the best diet to recommend to his or her patients. While it is relatively easy to tell everyone to eat a balanced diet of organically grown whole foods in as natural a form as possible, this ignores the biochemical uniqueness of each individual. Genetic and environmental factors dramatically alter a person's metabolism and without ways of objectively assessing these changes, all a physician can do is guess or blindly apply the latest theory. Over the centuries, many theories about how to optimize one's diet have come and gone, but none has survived the test of time, for none has been based on scientific research. Thanks to the pioneering work of Dr. Peter D'Adamo, and his father, Dr. James D'Adamo, this has now changed. Here is testimony to the fact that original ideas combined with a rigorous scientific perspective can change the course of medicine.

Joseph Pizzorno, N.D.
Seattle, Washington
June 1996

Dr. Pizzorno, President of Bastyr University in Seattle, Washington, the first accredited, multidisciplinary college of natural medicine in the United States, is a leading figure in the field of natural medicine. As senior editor and co-author of the internationally ac-

claimed A Textbook of Natural Medicine, *and the bestseller* Encyclopedia of Natural Medicine, *he helped define the standard of care for naturopathic medicine, documented the scientific validity of natural medicine, and pushed forward the frontiers of natural healing.*

In 1993, Dr. Pizzorno was invited to make a presentation on the role of naturopathic medicine in health care to First Lady Hillary Clinton's Health Care Reform Task Force. He was appointed to the U.S. Congress's Office of Technology Assessments Advisory Panel on the safety and efficacy of dietary supplements, and became a consultant to the U.S. Federal Trade Commission.

Blood Type Charts

Type O

The Hunter

strong
self-reliant
leader

STRENGTHS	WEAKNESSES	MEDICAL RISKS	DIET PROFILE	WEIGHT-LOSS KEY	SUPPLEMENTS	EXERCISE REGIMEN
Hardy digestive tract	Intolerant to new dietary, environment conditions	Blood-clotting disorders	High protein: Meat eaters	Avoid: wheat corn kidney beans	vitamin B vitamin K calcium iodine licorice kelp	Intense physical exercise, such as:
Strong immune system		Inflammatory diseases— arthritis	meat fish vegetables fruit	navy beans lentils cabbage		*aerobics *martial arts *contact sports
Natural defenses against infections	Immune system can be *over*active and attack itself	Low thyroid production	Limited: grains, beans, legumes	Brussels sprouts cauliflower mustard greens		*running
System designed for efficient metabolism and preservation of nutrients		Ulcers Allergies		Aids: kelp seafood salt liver red meat kale spinach broccoli		

T_{ype} A

The Cultivator

settled
cooperative
orderly

STRENGTHS	WEAKNESSES	MEDICAL RISKS	DIET PROFILE	WEIGHT-LOSS KEY	SUPPLEMENTS	EXERCISE REGIMEN
Adapts well to dietary and environmental changes	Sensitive digestive tract	Heart disease	Vegetarian	Avoid:	vitamin B-12	Calming, centering exercises, such as:
			vegetables	meat		
			tofu	dairy		
		Cancer	seafood	kidney beans	folic acid	
	Vulnerable		grains	lima beans	vitamin C	*Yoga
Immune	immune system,	Anemia	beans	wheat		
system preserves	open to microbial	Liver and gallbladder	legumes fruit	Aids:	vitamin E	*Tai chi
and metabolizes	invasion	disorders		vegetable oil	hawthorn	
nutrients more		Type I		soy foods vegetables	echinacea	
easily		Diabetes		pineapple	quercitin	
					milk thistle	

Type B

The Nomad

---

balanced
flexible
creative

STRENGTHS	WEAKNESSES	MEDICAL RISKS	DIET PROFILE	WEIGHT-LOSS KEY	SUPPLEMENTS	EXERCISE REGIMEN
Strong immune system	No natural weaknesses, but	Type I diabetes	Balanced omnivore	Avoid: corn lentil peanuts sesame seeds buckwheat wheat	magnesium	Moderate physical, with mental balance— such as:
Versatile adaptation to dietary and environmental changes	imbalance causes tendency toward autoimmune breakdowns and rare viruses	Chronic fatigue syndrome Autoimmune disorders— Lou Gehrig's disease, lupus, multiple sclerosis	meat (No chicken) dairy grains beans legumes vegetables fruit	Aids: greens eggs venison liver licorice tea	licorice ginkgo lecithin	*hiking *cycling *tennis *swimming
Balanced nervous system						

Type AB

The Enigma

---

r a r e
c h a r i s m a t i c
m y s t e r i o u s

STRENGTHS	WEAKNESSES	MEDICAL RISKS	DIET PROFILE	WEIGHT-LOSS KEY	SUPPLEMENTS	EXERCISE REGIMEN
Designed for modern conditions	Sensitive digestive tract	Heart disease	Mixed diet in moderation	Avoid: red meat kidney beans	vitamin C hawthorn	Calming, centering exercises, such as:
Highly tolerant immune system	Tendency for over-tolerant immune system, allowing microbial invasion	Cancer Anemia	meat seafood dairy tofu beans legumes grains vegetables fruit	lima beans seeds corn buckwheat	echinacea valerian quercitin	*Yoga *Tai chi
Combines benefits of Type A and Type B				Aids: tofu seafood dairy greens kelp pineapple	milk thistle	Com-bined with moderate physical such as:
	Reacts negatively to A-like and B-like conditions					*hiking *cycling *tennis

Common
Questions

IT HAS BEEN MY EXPERIENCE THAT MOST PEOPLE RESPOND with great enthusiasm and curiosity when they learn about the blood type connection. Yet it is far easier to embrace a provocative idea than it is to immerse oneself in the gritty details.

The Blood Type Plan is revolutionary, and as such requires many fundamental adjustments. Some people find it easier than others, depending on how much they're already living according to the needs of their blood type. Most of the questions people ask me have similar themes. I've included the most common ones here. They may help you get a clearer sense of what this diet will mean for you.

Where does my blood type come from?

Blood is universal, yet it is also unique. Like the color of your eyes or hair, your blood type is determined by two sets of genes—the inheritance you receive from your mother and father. It is from those genes commingling that your blood type is selected, at the moment of your conception.

Like genes, some blood types are dominant over others. In the cellular creation of a new human being, Type A and Type B are dominant over Type O. If at conception the embryo is given an A gene from the mother and an O gene from the father, the infant will be Type A, although it will continue to carry the father's O gene unexpressed in its DNA. When the infant grows up and passes these genes to its offspring, half of the genes will be for Type A blood and half will be for Type O blood.

Because A and B genes are equally strong, you are Type AB if you received an A gene from one parent and a B gene from the other. Finally, because the O gene is recessive to all the others, you are Type O only if you receive an O gene from each parent.

It is possible for two Type A parents to conceive a child who is Type O. This happens when the parents each have one A gene and one O gene and both pass the O gene on to the offspring. In the same way two brown-eyed parents can conceive a blue-eyed offspring if each carries the sleeping recessive gene for blue eyes.

Blood type genetics can sometimes be used to help determine the paternity of a child. There is one catch, however. Blood type can only prove that a man is not the father of a child. It cannot be used to prove that a man *is* the child's father (although newer DNA technology can do that). Consider this example, a paternity case: An infant is Type A, the mother is Type O, and the man alleged to be the father is Type B. As both A and B genes are dominant to O, the child's father could not be Type B. Think about it. The child's A gene could not have come from the father, who, because he was Type B, would have either two B genes or a B gene and an O gene. Nor could the A gene come from the mother, because people with Type O blood always carry two O genes. The A gene had to come from someone else. These were the exact circumstances surrounding the famous paternity suit against Charlie Chaplin in 1944. Unfortunately, Chaplin was subjected to a tumultuous trial, because the use of blood type to determine paternity was not yet acceptable in a California court of law. Even though blood type had clearly shown that Chaplin was not the father of the child, the jury still decided in favor of the mother, and he was forced to pay child support.

How do I find out my blood type?

To find out your blood type, you can donate blood, or you can call your doctor to see if your blood type is in your medical file. If you'd like to test your own blood type, you can do so by ordering a finger-stick test from the following address:

Peter D'Adamo, N.D.
P.O. Box 2106
Norwalk, CT 06852-2106

Do I have to make all of the changes at once for my Blood Type Diet to work?

No. On the contrary, I suggest you start slowly, gradually eliminating the foods that are not good for you, and increasing those that are highly beneficial. Many diet programs urge you to plunge in headfirst and radically change your lifestyle immediately. I think it's more realistic and ultimately more effective if you engage in a learning process. Don't just take my word for it. You have to learn it in your body.

Before you begin your Blood Type Diet, you may know very little about which foods are good or bad for you. You're used to making your choices according to your taste buds, family traditions, and fad diet books. Chances are you are eating some foods that are good for you, but the Blood Type Diet provides you with a powerful tool for making informed choices every time.

Once you know what your optimal eating plan is, you have the freedom to veer from your diet on occasion. Rigidity is the enemy of joy; I certainly am not a proponent of it. The Blood Type Diet is designed to make you feel great, not miserable and deprived. Obviously, there are going to be times when common sense tells you to relax the rules a bit—like when you're eating at a relative's house.

I'm Blood Type A and my husband is Blood Type O. How do we cook and eat together? I don't want to prepare two separate meals.

My wife, Martha, and I have exactly the same situation. Martha is Type O and I am Type A. We find that we can usually share about two-thirds of a meal. The main difference is in the protein source. For example, if we make a stir-fry, Martha might separately prepare some chicken, while I'll add cooked tofu. We have also found that many Type O and Type A foods are beneficial for both of us, so we emphasize those foods. For example, we might have a meal that includes salmon, rice, and broccoli. It has become relatively easy for us because we are quite familiar with the specifics of each other's Blood Type Diet. It will help you to spend some time getting familiar with your spouse's food lists. You can even make a separate list of foods that you can share. You might be surprised at how many there are.

People worry a lot about what they fear will be impossible limitations on the Blood Type Diet. But think about it. There are more than two hundred foods listed for each diet—many of them compatible across the board. Considering that the average person eats only about twenty-five foods, the Blood Type Diets actually offer more, not fewer, options.

My family is Italian, and you know the kinds of foods we like to eat. Being Type A, I don't see how I can still enjoy my favorite Italian foods—especially, no tomato sauce!

We tend to associate ethnic foods with one or two of the most commonly available—like spaghetti with meat balls and tomato sauce. But the Italian diet, like most others, includes a wide variety of different foods. Many southern Italian dishes, usually prepared with olive oil instead of heavy sauces, are wonderful choices for both Type A and Type AB. Instead of a plate of pasta drenched in red sauce, try the more delicate flavors of olive oil and garlic, a complex pesto, or a light white wine sauce. Fresh fruits or flavorful but light Italian ices are preferable to rich pastries.

My seventy-year-old husband has a history of heart problems, and has had bypass surgery. He still has a hard time staying away from the wrong foods. He's Type B and I think the Type B Diet would be perfect for him. But he's very resistant to diets. Is there a good way to introduce the diet without a lot of fuss?

It isn't easy to radically change your diet at age seventy—which is probably why your husband has had so much trouble eating healthily, even after surgery. Rather than nagging, which is usually counterproductive, begin to gradually incorporate the beneficial Type B foods into his diet, while slowly eliminating those that aren't good for Type Bs. It's likely that your husband will develop preferences for the good foods as his digestive tract adjusts to their positive qualities.

Why do you list different portion recommendations according to ancestry?

The portion listings according to ancestry are merely refinements to the diet that you may find helpful. In the same way that men, women, and children have different portion standards, so too do people according to their body size and weight, geography, and cultural food preferences. These suggestions will help you until you are comfortable enough with the diet to naturally eat the appropriate portions.

The portion recommendations also take into account specific problems that people of different ancestries tend to have with food. African-Americans, for example, are often lactose intolerant, and most Asians are unaccustomed to eating dairy foods, so they may have to introduce these foods slowly to avoid negative reactions.

I'm allergic to peanuts, but you say they're a highly beneficial food for my blood type. Are you saying I should eat them? I'm Type A.

No. Type As have plenty of great protein sources without peanuts. These reactions are generated by the immune system, which creates antibodies that resist the food. Chances are, a person with Type A blood would not be allergic to peanuts, which contain friendly, A-like properties. You may, however, be intolerant to peanuts. That means you have digestive distress when you eat them. This could be caused by any number of factors, including an overall poor diet. Maybe you once ate peanuts, along with other problem foods, and blamed the peanuts.

Again, you don't need to include peanuts in your diet, but you may find that you tolerate them quite well once you've adjusted to the Type A Diet.

I'm Type B and my meat choices are very strange to me. It looks as though all I can eat are lamb, mutton, venison, and rabbit—which I NEVER eat. Why no chicken?

The elimination of chicken is the toughest adjustment for most people I've treated who are Type B. Not only is chicken a protein staple of many ethnic groups, but most of us have been conditioned to think that chicken is healthier than beef and other meats. Once again, however, there is no single rule that works for everyone. Chicken contains a lectin in its muscle meat that is very detrimental to Type Bs. On the brighter side, you can eat turkey and a wide variety of seafood.

What does "neutral" mean? Are these foods good for me?

The three categories are designed to focus on the foods which are most and least beneficial to you, according to your blood type reaction to certain lectins. The highly beneficial foods act as a medicine; the foods to avoid act as a poison. The neutral foods simply act as foods. While the neutral foods may not have the special health benefits of some other foods, they're certainly good for you in the sense that they contain many nutrients that your body needs.

Must I eat all of the foods marked "highly beneficial"?

It would be impossible to eat everything on your diet! Think of your Blood Type Diet as a painter's palette from which you may choose colors in different shades and combinations. However, do try to reach the weekly amount of the various food groups if possible. Frequency is probably more important than the individual portion sizes, so if you are Type O and have a very small build, try to have animal protein five to seven times weekly, but cut back on the portions, perhaps using two to three ounces instead of four to five ounces. This ensures that the most valuable nutrients will continue to be delivered into the bloodstream at a constant rate.

Is food combining helpful on the Blood Type Diet?

Some diet plans recommend food combining, which involves eating certain food groups in combination for better digestion. Many of these books are full of bunk and hokum, with a lot of unnecessary rules and regulations. Perhaps the only real food-combining rule is to avoid eating animal proteins, such as meats, with large amounts of starches, such as breads and potatoes. This is important because animal products are digested in the stomach in a high-acid environment, while starches are digested in the intestines in a high-alkaline environment. When these foods are combined, the body alternately nibbles at the protein, then the starch, then back to the protein, then back to the starch; not a very efficient method. By keeping these food groups separated, the stomach can concentrate its full functions on the job at hand. Substitute low-starch, high-fiber vegetable side dishes, such as greens. Protein-starch avoidance doesn't apply to tofu and other vegetable proteins, which are essentially predigested.

What should I do if a "food to avoid" is the fourth or fifth ingredient in a recipe?

That depends on the severity of your condition, or the degree of your compliance. If you have food allergies, or colitis, you may want to practice complete avoidance. Many high-compliance patients avoid these foods altogether, although I think this might be too extreme. Unless they suffer from a specific allergic condition, it won't hurt most people to occasionally eat a food that is not on their diet.

Will I lose weight on the Blood Type Diet?

When you read your Blood Type Plan, you will find specific recommendations for weight loss. They differ from blood type to blood type. That's because the lectins in various foods have a different effect. For example, for Type O, meat is efficiently digested and metabolized, while for Type A it slows the digestive and metabolic processes.

Your Blood Type Diet is tailor made to eliminate any imbalances that lead to weight gain. If you follow your Blood Type Diet, your metabolism will adjust to its normal level and you'll burn calories more efficiently; your digestive system will process nutrients properly and reduce water retention. You'll lose weight immediately.

In my practice, I've found that most of my patients who have weight problems also have a history of chronic dieting. One would think that constant dieting would lead to weight loss, but that's not true if the structure of the diet and the foods it includes go against everything that makes sense for your specific body.

In our culture, we tend to promote "one size fits all" weight-loss programs, and then we wonder why they don't work. The answer is obvious! Different blood types respond to food in different ways. In conjunction with the recommended exercise program, you should see results very quickly.

Do calories matter on the Blood Type Diet?

As with most general diet issues, concerns about calories are automatically taken care of by following your specific Blood Type Diet. Most new patients who follow the guidelines concerning diet and exercise lose some weight. Some people even complain that they are losing too much weight. There is an adjustment period on this diet, and over time you'll be able to find the food amounts that suit your needs. However, the charts in each food category give you a place to start.

It's important to be aware of portion sizes. No matter what you eat, if you eat too much of it you'll gain weight. This probably seems so obvious that it doesn't even bear mentioning. But overeating has become one of America's most difficult and dangerous health problems. Millions of Americans are bloated and dyspeptic because of the amounts of food they eat. When you eat excessively, the walls of your stomach stretch like an inflated balloon. Although stomach muscles are elastic and were created to contract and expand, when they are grossly enlarged the cells of the abdominal walls undergo a tremendous strain. If you are eating until you feel full, and you normally feel sluggish after a meal, try to reduce your portion sizes. Learn to listen to what your body is telling you.

I have heart problems and I've been told to totally avoid any fat and cholesterol. I'm Type O. How can I eat meat?

First, realize that it is grains, not meats, which are the cardiovascular culprits for Type O. This is especially interesting because almost everybody who has or is attempting to prevent heart disease is advised to go on a diet based largely on complex carbohydrates!

For Type Os, a high intake of certain carbohydrates, usually wheat breads, increases the insulin levels. In response, your body stores more fat in the tissues, and fat levels are elevated in the blood.

Also bear in mind that your blood cholesterol level is only moderately controlled by the dietary intake of foods that are high in cholesterol content. Approximately 85 to 90 percent is actually controlled by the manufacture and metabolism of cholesterol in your liver.

I'm Type O and don't want to eat much fat in my diet. What do you suggest?

A high-protein diet does not automatically mean one that is high in fat, especially if you avoid heavily marbleized meats. Although more expensive, try to find free-range meats that have been raised without the excessive use of antibiotics and other chemicals. Our ancestors consumed rather lean game or domestic animals that grazed on alfalfa and other grasses; today's high-fat meats are produced by using high amounts of corn feed.

If you can't afford or can't find free-range meats, choose the leanest cuts available and remove all excess fat before cooking. Type Os also have many other good protein choices that are naturally lower in fat—such as chicken and seafood. The fat in the oil-rich fish is composed of omega-3 fatty acids, which seem to promote lower cholesterol and healthier hearts.

How can I be sure to buy the most natural and the freshest foods?

Within the last few years, many consumers have banded together to create food co-ops, groups of people who buy in bulk. Very often this bulk purchasing power results in great savings and high-quality produce. Most food co-ops require a small membership fee and a few hours of work at the co-op per month. Savings, especially on items such as grains, spices, beans, vegetables, and oils can be substantial.

Health food stores can be a valuable place to buy fresh foods, but don't fall into the trap of thinking that because you are in a health food store you can relax your guard. Many health food stores, especially the smaller ones, do not have the rapid turnover of a busy greengrocer or supermarket, and their foods might not be as fresh.

Are organic foods more healthy than non-organic foods?

A good rule of thumb is to use organic vegetables if they are not exorbitantly priced. They do taste better, and are more healthy. However, if you are on a fixed income and cannot find competitively priced organic produce, high-quality, properly cleaned, fresh non-organic produce will do just fine.

More and more supermarkets seem to be stocking organic produce, mostly from California, a state with specific laws concerning the use of the term *organic*. Interestingly, in one supermarket in my neighborhood, organic vegetables and fruits are displayed next to the non-organic versions, and are priced identically! I suspect that market pressures will continue to push more and more vegetable and fruit growers toward the organic way, if for no other reason than the cost of commercial fertilizers, made from petrochemicals, will eventually make them more expensive to produce than naturally grown products.

Will eating canned food hurt my diet?

Commercially canned foods, subject to high heat and pressure, lose most of their vitamin content, especially the antioxidants, such as vitamin C. They do retain the vitamins that are not heat sensitive, such as vitamin A. Canned foods typically are lower in fiber than their fresh counterparts and higher in salt, usually added to offset the loss of flavors in production. Soggy, with little of the "life" we find in fresh foods and vegetables, and few natural enzymes (which are destroyed by the canning process), canned foods should be used sparingly, if at all. You pay much more per weight for canned food, and don't get back much in return.

Other than fresh, frozen foods are your best second bet. Freezing does not change the nutritional content of the food very much (its preparation before freezing may) although the taste and texture are often blunted.

Why is stir-frying so beneficial?

The quick frying of Oriental-style cooking is healthier than deep frying. Less oil is used, and the oil itself, typically sesame oil, is more resistant to high temperatures than safflower or canola oils. The idea behind stir-frying is to quickly braise the food on its outside, which has the added effect of sealing in flavors.

Most types of meals can be prepared in this manner using a wok. The deep, cone-shaped design of the wok concentrates the heat at a small area at its base, which allows food to be cooked there and then moved to the cooler edges of the pan. Wok cooking usually mixes vegetables and seafoods or meats. Cook the meats and vegetables that require longer heating first, then move them to the outside of the pan, adding the vegetables that require less cooking to the center.

Steaming vegetables is also a quick and effective method of cooking, and helps to keep the nutrients in the food. Use a simple steamer basket, purchased at any hardware or department store, fitted inside a large pot filled with water to the level of the basket bottom. Add vegetables, cover and heat. Don't cook until soggy! Crisp means better taste, better texture, and better nutrition.

Should I take a multivitamin every day on the Blood Type Diet?

If you are in good health and are following your Blood Type Diet, you shouldn't really need a supplement, although there are exceptions. Pregnant women should supplement their diet with iron, calcium, and folic acid. Most women also need extra calcium—especially if their diet doesn't include many dairy foods.

Those engaged in heavy physical activity, people in stressful occupations, the elderly, those who are ill, heavy smokers—all should be on a supplementation program. More specific details are available in your individual Blood Type Plan.

How important are herbs and herbal teas?

That depends on your blood type. Type Os respond well to soothing herbs, Type As to the more stimulating ones, and Type Bs do quite nicely without most of them. Type ABs should follow the herbal protocols laid down for Type As, with the added proviso that Type ABs shun those herbs that both Type As and Type Bs are asked to avoid.

Why are vegetable oils so limited on the Blood Type Diet? I thought all vegetable oils were good for you.

What you've probably heard is advertisers hawking the news that vegetable oils have "No Cholesterol!" Well, that's not news to anyone with even a modicum of knowledge about nutrition. Plants and vegetables do not manufacture cholesterol, which is found only in products derived from animals. Your cholesterol-free oil may have little else to recommend it.

Here are the facts. Always avoid tropical oils, such as coconut oil, as they are high in saturated fat, which can be harmful to the cardiovascular system. Most oils sold today, including safflower and canola (rapeseed) are polyunsaturated, which makes them an improvement over lard and tropical oils. However, there is some concern that overconsumption of polyunsaturated fats may be linked to certain types of cancer, especially if they're subjected to the high temperatures of cooking. In general, I prefer to use olive oil as much as possible in cooking. I believe that olive oil has proven to be the most tolerated and beneficial of fats. As a monounsaturated oil it seems to have positive effects on the heart and arteries. There are many different blends of olive oil available. The finest quality is the extra-virgin grade. It is slightly greenish in color and almost odorless—although when gently heated, the perfume of the olives is sensational. Olive oil is usually cold-pressed rather than extracted using heat or chemicals. The less processed an oil is, the better its quality.

Tofu seems like a very unappealing food. Must I eat it if I'm Type A?

Many Type A and Type AB people raise their eyebrows and grimace with disgust when I recommend that they make tofu a staple of their diets. Well, tofu is not a glamour food. I admit it.

When I was an impoverished Type A college student, I ate tofu with vegetables and brown rice almost every day for years. It was cheap, but I actually liked it.

I think the real problem with tofu is the way it is usually displayed in the markets. Tofu—in soft or hard cakes—sits with its other tofu friends in a large plastic tub, immersed in cold water. When people manage to overcome their initial aversion and actually purchase one or two tofu cakes (calling them cakes has a rather bitter irony), many people take it home, pop it on a plate, and break off a hunk to give it a try. This is a bad way to experience tofu! It might be comparable to tossing a whole raw egg into your mouth and chewing . . . not a very pleasant experience.

If you are going to use tofu, it is best cooked and combined with vegetables and strong flavors that you enjoy, such as garlic, ginger, and soy sauce.

Tofu is a nutritionally complete meal that is filling and extremely inexpensive. Type As take note: The path to your good health is paved with bean curd!

I've never heard of many of the grains you mention. Where do I find out more?

If you're looking for alternative grains, health food stores are a bonanza. In recent years, many ancient grains, largely forgotten, have been rediscovered and are now being produced. Examples of these are amaranth, a grain from Mexico, and spelt, a variation of wheat that seems to be free of the problems found with whole wheat. Try them! They're not bad. Spelt flour makes a hearty, chewy bread that is quite flavorful, while several interesting breakfast cereals are now being made with amaranth. Another alternative is to use sprouted-wheat breads, sometimes referred to as Ezekiel or Essene bread, as the gluten lectins found principally in the seed coat are destroyed by the sprouting process. These breads spoil rapidly and are usually found in the refrigerator cases of health food stores. They are a live food, with many beneficial enzymes still intact. Beware of commercially produced sprouted wheat breads, as they usually have a minority of sprouted wheat and a majority of whole wheat in their formulas. Sprouted bread is somewhat sweet tasting, as the sprouting process also releases sugars, and it is moist and chewy. This bread makes wonderful toast.

I'm type A and I've been a runner for many years. Running seems to be a great way to reduce stress. I'm confused about your advice that I shouldn't exercise heavily.

There is a great deal of evidence that your blood type informs your unique reaction to stress, and that Type As tend to do better with less intense exercise. My father has observed this thousands of times in his thirty-five years studying the connection. However, there is much we don't yet know, so I would hesitate to say absolutely that you shouldn't run.

I would ask you to reevaluate your health and energy levels. I often have patients who say things like, "I've always been a runner," or "I've always eaten chicken," as if that were all the proof they needed that an activity or a food was beneficial. Often, these very people are suffering from an assortment of physical problems and stresses that they've never thought to associate with specific activities or foods. You may be a Type A with a twist—one who thrives on intense physical activity. Or you may discover that you're running on empty.

Glossary
of Terms

ABO BLOOD GROUP SYSTEM: THE MOST IMPORTANT OF THE blood-typing systems, the ABO blood group is the determinant for transfusion reactions and organ transplantation. Unlike the other blood-typing systems, the ABO blood types have far-ranging significance other than transfusion or transplantation, including the determination of many of the digestive and immunological characteristics of the body. The ABO blood group is comprised of four blood types: O, A, B and AB. Type O has no true antigen, but carries antibodies to both A and B blood. Type A and type B carry the antigen named for their blood type and make antibodies to each other. Type AB does not manufacture any antibodies to other blood types because it has both A and B antigens.

Anthropologists use the ABO blood types extensively as a guide to the development of early peoples. Many diseases, especially digestive disorders, cancer, and infection, express preferences, choosing between the ABO blood types. These expressions are not generally understood or appreciated by either physicians or the general population.

Agglutinate: Derived from the Latin word "to glue." The process by which cells are made to adhere to one another, usually through the actions of an agglutinin, such as an antibody or a lectin. Certain viruses and bacteria also are capable of agglutinating blood cells. Many agglutinins, particularly the food lectins, are blood type specific. Certain foods clump only the cells of one blood type, but do not react with the cells of another type.

Anthropology: The study of the human race in relation to distribution, origin, and classification. Anthropologists study physical characteristics, the relationship of races, environmental and social relations, and culture. The ABO blood types are extensively used by anthropologists in the study of early human populations.

Antibody: A class of chemicals, called the immunoglobulins, made by the cells of the immune system to specifically tag or identify foreign material within the body of the host. Antibodies combine with specific markers—antigens—found on viruses, bacteria, or other toxins, and agglutinate them. The immune system is capable of manufacturing millions of different antibodies against a wide variety of potential invaders. Individuals of Type O, Type A, or Type B blood carry antibodies to other blood types. Type AB, the universal recipient, manufactures no antibodies to other types.

Antigen: Any chemical that generates an antibody by the immune system in response to it. The chemical markers which determine blood type are considered blood type antigens because other blood types may carry antibodies to them. Antigens are commonly found on the surface of germs, and are used by the immune system to detect foreign material. Specialized antigens are often made by cancer cells, these being called tumor antigens. Many germs and cancer antigens are clever impersonators who can mimic the blood type of the host in an effort to escape detection.

Antioxidant: Vitamins that are believed to strengthen the immune system and prevent cancer by fighting off toxic compounds (called free radicals) that attack cells. Vitamins C, E, and beta-carotene are believed to be the most powerful antioxidants.

Cro-Magnon: The first truly modern human. Originating around 70,000 to 40,000 B.C., Cro-Magnon migrated extensively from Africa into Europe and Asia. A master hunter, Cro-Magnon led a largely hunter-gatherer existence. Most of the digestive characteristics of people with Type O blood are derived from Cro-Magnon.

Differentiation: The cellular process by which cells develop their specialized characteristics and functions. Differentiation is controlled by the genetic machinery of the cell. Cancer cells, which often have defective genes, usually de-evolve, and lose many of the characteristics of a normal cell, often reverting to earlier embryologic forms long re-pressed since early development.

Gene: A component of the cell that controls the transmission of hereditary characteristics by specifying the construction of a particular protein or enzyme. Genes are composed of long chains of de-oxyribonucleic acid (DNA) contained in the chromosomes of the cell nucleus.

Indo-European: An early Caucasian people who migrated westward to Europe from their early homelands in Asia and the Middle East around 7000 to 3500 B.C. The Indo-Europeans were probably the progenitors for Type A blood in western Europe.

Ketosis: A state that is achieved with a high-protein, low-carbohydrate diet. The high-protein diets of our early Type O ancestors forced the burning of fat for energy and the production of ketones—a sign of rapid metabolic activity. The state of ketosis allowed early humans to maintain high energy, metabolic efficiency, and physical strength—all qualities needed for hunting game.

Lectin: Any compound, usually a protein, found in nature, which can interact with surface antigens found on the body's cells, causing them to agglutinate. Lectins are often found in common foods, and many of them are blood type specific. Because cancer cells often manufacture copious amounts of antigens on their surface, many lectins will agglutinate them in preference to normal cells.

Mucus: Secretions manufactured by specialized tissues, called mucous membranes, which are used to lubricate and protect the delicate internal linings of the body. Mucus contains antibodies to protect against germs. In secretors, large amounts of blood type antigens are secreted in mucus, which serves to filter out bacteria, fungi, and parasites with opposing blood type characteristics.

Naturopathic doctor (N.D.): A physician trained in natural healing methods. Naturopathic doctors receive a four-year postgraduate training at an accredited college or university, and function as primary-care providers.

Neolithic: The period of early human development characterized by the development of agriculture and the use of pottery and polished tools. The radical change in human lifestyle, from the previous hunter-gatherer existence, probably was a major stimulus to the development of Blood Type A.

Panhemaglutinans: Lectins that agglutinate all blood types. An example is the tomato lectin.

Polymorphism: Literally means "many shapes." A polymorphism is any physical manifestation between a species of living organisms which is variable through genetic influence. The blood types are a well-known polymorphism.

Phytochemical: Any natural product with specific health applications. Most phytochemicals are traditional herbs and plants.

Triglycerides: The body's fat stores, also contained in the bloodstream. High tryglycerides—or high blood fats—are considered a risk for heart disease.

Notes on the Anthropology of Blood Type

ANTHROPOLOGY IS THE STUDY OF HUMAN DIFFERENCES, cultural and biological. Most anthropologists divide the field into two categories: cultural anthropology, which looks at the manifestations of culture, such as language or ritual; and physical anthropology, the study of the evolutionary biology of our species, *Homo sapiens*. Physical anthropologists attempt to trace human historical development through hard scientific methods, such as the blood types. A central task in physical anthropology has been to document the sequence of how the human line evolved from early primate ancestors. The use of blood types to study early societies has been termed paleoserology, the study of ancient blood.

Physical anthropology is also concerned with how humans adapted to environmental pressures. Traditional physical anthropology relied heavily on the measuring of skull shape, stature, and other physical characteristics. Blood type became a powerful tool for this type of analysis. In the 1950s, as emphasis shifted to genetic characteristics, interest shifted to the blood types and other markers that have known genetic bases. A. E. Mourant, a physician and anthropologist, has published two key works, *Blood Groups and Disease* (1978), and *Blood Relations: Blood Groups and Anthropology* (1985), which have collected much of the available material on the subject.

In addition to Mourant, I've used a variety other source material for this appendix, including earlier anthropology sources such as William Boyd's *Genetics and the Races of Man* (1950), and a series of studies that were published in various journals of forensic medicine from 1920 to 1945.

It is possible to map the occurrence of the various blood groups in ancient populations by blood typing grave exhumations. Small amounts of blood type materials can be reconstituted from the remains, and the blood type determined. By studying the blood types of human populations, anthropologists gain information about that population's local history; movement, intermarriage, and diversification.

Many national and ethnic groups have unique blood type distributions. In certain more isolated cultures, a clear majority of one blood type over another can still be seen. In other societies, the distribution may be more even. In the United States, for example, the equal rates of Type O and Type A blood reflect masses of immigration. The United States also has a higher percentage of Blood Type B than the western European countries, which probably reflects the influx of more eastern nationalities.

For the purpose of this analysis, we can divide humankind into two basic races—Ethiopian and Palearctic. The Palearctic can be further broken down to Mongolians and Caucasians, although most people lie somewhere in between. Each race is physically characterized by its environment and occupies distinct geographic areas. Ethiopians, probably the oldest race, are dark-skinned Africans, inhabiting the southern third of Arabia and sub-Saharan Africa. The Palearctic region comprises Africa north of the Sahara, then Europe, most of Asia (with the exception of southern Arabia), India, Southeast Asia, and southern China.

The roughest guesswork places the beginnings of human migration from Africa to Asia at about 1 million years ago. In Asia, most likely, modern *Homo sapiens* species split from a trunk of the ancestral Ethiopians into the Caucasians and Mongolians, but we know almost nothing about when or why it occurred.

Each of the basic races has its own homeland—a geographic area where it is preeminent. The Ethiopian homeland was Africa, the Caucasian Europe and northern Asia, and the Mongolian central and southern Asia.

As human groups migrated and interbred, intermediate populations evolved in the creases and crevices between these ancestral homelands. The area bound by the Sahara, the Middle East, and Somalia, for example, was home to a blending of the African and Caucasian races; the Indian subcontinent, a blend of the more northerly Caucasians and the more southerly Mongolians. These groups, which then split into innumerable, often temporary populations, were subject to the pressures of disease, food sources, and climate. They may have existed for thousands of years in the spaces between the homelands. Although the result of migration was to spread Type O blood far and wide around the world, it was from these spaces that the later blood types emerged.

There may be more physical differences between Africans and the other races, but the blood type differences between Caucasians and Mongolians are more clear cut—a good reason to re-examine racial stereotypes.

It would also be a mistake to think of the early Type O people as primitives. More intellectual development occurred in the Cro-Magnon age than in any time before or after. The Cro-Magnons created our early societies and rituals, more than the rudiments of communication, and the original wanderlust. Although we trace the genetic heritage of Type O blood back to early prehistory, it still remains a very workable chemistry, largely because of its simplicity and the fact that animal protein diets still account for a great portion of the world's current food intake.

The first attempt at using blood type to describe racial and nationality characteristics was undertaken by a husband-and-wife team of physicians, the Hirszfelds, in 1918. During the First World War both had served as doctors in the Allied armies that had concentrated in the area of Salonika, Greece.

Working with a multinational force, and with large amounts of refugees of different ethnic backgrounds, the Hirszfelds systematically blood-typed large numbers of people while also recording their race and nationality. Each group contained over five hundred or more subjects.

They found, for example, that the rate of Blood Type B ranged from a low of 7.2 percent of the population of English subjects, to a high of 41.2 percent in Indians, and that western Europeans in general had a lower incidence of Type B than Balkan Slavs, who had a lower incidence than Russians, Turks, and Jews; who again had a lower occurrence than Vietnamese and Indians. The distribution of Blood Type AB essentially followed the same pattern, with a low of 3 to 5 percent in western Europeans, and a high of 8.5 percent in Indians.

In subcontinental India, Type ABs make up 8.5 percent of the population—remarkably high for a blood type that averages between 2 and 5 percent worldwide. This prevalence of Type ABs is probably due to subcontinental India's location as an invasion route between the conquered lands to the west and the Mongolian homelands to the east.

Blood Type O and Type A were essentially the reverse of Type B and Type AB. The percentage of Type A remained fairly consistent (40 percent) among Europeans, Balkan Slavs, and Arabs, while being quite low in west Africans, Vietnamese, and Indians. Forty-six percent of the English population tested were Type O, which accounted for only 31.3 percent of the Indians tested.

Modern analysis (largely the result of records kept by blood banks), encompasses the blood types of more than 20 million individuals from around the world. Yet these large numbers can do no more than confirm the original observations of the Hirszfelds. No scientific journals saw fit to publish their material at that time. For a while, the Hirszfelds' study languished in an obscure anthropology journal; for more than thirty years this fascinating and important work was overlooked.

Apparently, there was little interest in using this knowledge of the blood types as an anthropological probe into the history of humanity.

Racial Classifications Based on Blood Type

IN THE 1920s several anthropologists first attempted racial classification based on blood groups. In 1929 Laurance Snyder published a book called *Blood Grouping in Relationship to Clinical and Legal Medicine*. In it, Snyder proposed a comprehensive classification system based on blood type. It is especially interesting because it focuses largely on the distribution of the ABO groups, the only tool to be had at the time.

The racial classifications—as Snyder saw them—were:

THE EUROPEAN TYPE: High frequency of Blood Type A, low frequency of Type B, perhaps the result of Type A blood originating in western Europe. This category included English, Scots, French, Belgians, Italians, and Germans.

INTERMEDIATE TYPE: A sort of blend between western (high Type A) and central (high Type B) European populations. Higher incidence of Blood Type O overall. This category included the Finns, Arabs, Russians, Spanish Jews, Armenians, and Lithuanians.

HUNAN TYPE: Oriental groups with a high incidence of Blood Type A, possibly the result of an infusion of Caucasian elements, including the Ukrainians, Poles, Hungarians, Japanese, Romanian Jews, Koreans, and southern Chinese.

INDOMANCHURIAN TYPE: Contain population groups with a high incidence of Blood Type B over Type A. This type includes the subcontinental Indians, Gypsies, Northern Chinese, and Manchus.

AFRICO-MALAYSIAN TYPE: Moderately higher incidence of Type A and Type B overall, with normal incidence of Type O. This category includes Javanese, Sumatrans, Africans, and Moroccans.

PACIFIC-AMERICAN TYPE: Including Filipinos, North and South American Indians, and Eskimos. Extremely high incidence of Type O and Rh+ blood types, very small incidence of Type A, and almost absent incidence of Type B.

AUSTRALASIAN TYPE: Principally the Australian Aborigines, this classification shows high incidence of Type A (almost equivalent to western Europe), almost no Type B, and a high incidence of Type O, although not as high as found with the Pacific American type.

Because he could only rely on ABO blood types, Snyder's classifications made for some strange pairings, such as the Hunan type containing both Koreans and Romanian Jews. Later, researchers began using the Rh and MN blood types, in addition to the ABO in their classifications, trying to refine these categories. They were aware that racial classification based merely on ABO groups would, in many cases, give results which would not coincide with older ideas about race, so they also incorporated MN types and occasional other blood factors (see Appendix E) to distinguish populations not clearly differentiated by ABO.

One classification, based on these newer criteria, distinguished the following races:

Europeans (Nordics and Alpines of Europe/Near East)
Mediterranean
Mongolian (Central Asia and Eurasia)
African
Indonesian
American Indian
Oceanic (including Japanese)
Australian

Another racial classification, based largely on ABO and Rh factors:

CAUCASIAN GROUP: Highest incidence of Rh−, relatively high Type A, moderately high incidence of all other blood types.

NEGROID GROUP: Highest incidence of rare Rh types, moderate frequency of Rh−, high relative incidence of Blood

Type A2, and the rare intermediates of Type A—Ax and A Bantu.

Mongolian group: Virtual absence of blood types Rh– and Type A2. Using MN data further classified the Mongolian group into the Asiatic group, Pacific Island and Australian group, American Indian and Eskimo group.

William Boyd, in his 1950 book *Genetics and the Races of Man*, proposed a more accurate classification based on this earlier classification:

Early European group: Possessing the highest incidence (over 30 percent) of the Rh–, and probably no Type B. A relatively high incidence of Blood Type O. The gene for subtype N possibly somewhat higher than in present-day Europeans. Represented today by their modern descendants, the Basques.

European (Caucasoid) group: Possessing the next-highest incidence of the Rh– gene and a relatively high incidence of Blood Type A2, with moderate frequencies of other blood group genes. Normal frequencies of the gene for subtype M.

African (Negroid) group: Possessing a tremendously high incidence of a rare Rh+ blood type gene, Rh0, and a moderate frequency of Rh–; relatively high incidence of Type A2 and the rare intermediate types of A, and a rather high incidence of Blood Type B.

Asiatic (Mongolian) group: Possessing high frequencies of Blood Type B, but little if any of the genes for Blood Type A2 and Rh–.

American Indian group: Possessing little or no Type A, and probably no Type B or Rh–. Very high rates of Blood Type O.

AUSTRALOID GROUP: Possessing high incidence of Blood Type Al, but not Type A2, or Rh–. High incidence of gene for N subtype.

Boyd's classification made more sense than the earlier classification systems, because it also fit the geographic distributions of the individual races more accurately.

Recent work by Dr. Luigi Cavalli-Sforza at Stanford University has tracked the genetic drift of the ancient human migrations, using even more sophisticated methods based on the new DNA technology. Many of his findings have confirmed the earlier observations of Mourant, the Hirszfelds, Snyder, and Boyd concerning the distribution of blood types worldwide.

The Blood Type Subgroups

MORE THAN 90 PERCENT OF ALL FACTORS ASSOCIATED with blood type are related to your major ABO type. There are, however, many minor blood subtypes, most of them playing insignificant roles. Of all the subtypes, only three will have any impact on your profile or affect your health and diet. I mention them only because they occasionally pop up as a useful refinement in your health plan. But let me stress: Knowing whether you are Type O, Type A, Type B, or Type AB is the only blood type information you really need.

The three subtypes that play minor roles are:

- SECRETOR/NON-SECRETOR STATUS
- RH POSITIVE (RH+) AND RH NEGATIVE (RH–)
- THE MN BLOOD GROUP SYSTEM

Secretors and Non-Secretors

ALTHOUGH EVERYONE carries a blood type antigen on their blood cells, some people also have blood type antigens that float around freely in their body secretions. These people are called secretors, because they secrete their blood type antigens into their saliva, mucus, sperm, and other body fluids. In addition to their blood, it's possible to learn the blood type of a secretor from these other fluids. Secretors comprise about 80 percent of the population, non-secretors 20 percent.

Secretor status has important implications in law enforcement.

A semen sample taken from a rape victim can be used to help convict the rapist if he is a secretor and his blood type matches the blood type identified in the semen. However, if he is in the small population of non-secretors, his blood type cannot be identified from any fluids except the blood.

People who do not secrete their blood type antigens in other fluids besides blood are called non-secretors. Being a secretor or a non-secretor is independent of your ABO blood type; it is controlled by a different gene. Thus one person could be a Type A secretor, and another a Type A non-secretor.

Because secretors have more places to put their blood type antigens, they have more blood type expression in their bodies than non-secretors. Finding out whether or not you are a secretor is as easy as finding out your ABO blood type. The most common way to determine secretor status involves testing saliva for the presence of blood type activity. It is not a common test, although there are several laboratories (listed in the back of the book) that will perform it for a small fee. I suggest that until you find out your secretor status for certain, play the numerical odds and assume you are a secretor.

If you are tested for secretor status, something called the Lewis System will probably be used. It's a quick-and-dirty way to identify secretors and non-secretors, and I mention it here only so you can recognize it if you see it on a blood type report.

In the Lewis System there are two possible antigens that can be produced, called Lewis a and Lewis b (not to be confused with the A and B of the ABO system), and their interplay determines your secretor status. LEWIS a+ b− equals non-secretor. LEWIS a− b+ equals secretor.

Positive or Negative

WHEN WE blood-type patients in my office, they almost immediately ask if they are negative or positive. Many people don't realize that this is an additional separate blood grouping called the

Rhesus, or Rh, system, and it really has nothing to do with your ABO blood type—although it does have one important ramification for pregnant women.

The Rh system is named for the rhesus monkey, a commonly used laboratory animal, in whose blood it was first discovered. For many years it remained a mystery to doctors why some women who had normal first pregnancies developed complications in their second and subsequent pregnancies, often resulting in miscarriage and even the death of the mother. In 1940, it was discovered (again by the amazing Dr. Landsteiner) that these women were carrying a different blood type than their babies, who took their blood type from the father. The babies were Rh+, meaning that they carried the Rh antigen on their blood cells. Their mothers were Rh−, which meant that this antigen was missing from their blood. Unlike the ABO system, in which the antibodies to other blood types develop from birth, Rh− people do not make an antibody to the Rh antigen unless they are first sensitized. This sensitization usually occurs when blood is exchanged between the mother and infant during birth, so the mother's immune system does not have enough time to react to the first baby. However, should a subsequent conception result in another Rh+ baby, the mother, now sensitized, will produce antibodies to the baby's blood type. Reactions to the Rh factor can occur only in Rh− women who conceive the children of Rh+ fathers. Rh+ women, 85 percent of the population, have nothing to worry about. Even though the Rh system doesn't figure prominently when it comes to diets or diseases, it is certainly a factor for childbearing women who are Rh−.

IF YOU HAVE	BUT DO NOT HAVE	YOU ARE
The Rh antigen	The anti-Rh antibody	Rh+
The anti-Rh antibody	The Rh antigen	Rh−

The MN Blood Group System

THE MN blood group system is virtually unknown because it is not a major factor in transfusions or organ transplants, and is of little interest in the day-to-day practice of medicine. This is deceiving, however, because a variety of diseases are associated with them—if only in a minor way.

In this system, a person can type out as MM, NN, or MN, depending upon whether his or her cells have only the M antigen (which would make them MM), the N antigen (NN), or both (MN). This system will pop up occasionally in our discussions, especially when we talk about cancer and heart disease. Around 28 percent of the population is typed as MM, 22 percent as NN, and 50 percent as MN.

IF YOU HAVE	BUT DO NOT HAVE	YOU ARE
The M antigen	The N antigen	Type MM
The N antigen	The M antigen	Type NN
The M and N antigens		Type MN

Your Blood Type Pedigree

These three subtype systems are often used in my office, and they are often a part of various lab panels in use by other doctors. Although you can find almost all of the information you will ever need simply by knowing your ABO type, these systems offer a further refinement that allows a much deeper understanding of your blood's characteristics.

This results in what I call the blood type pedigree, a string of letters that is a patient's profile. In many ways, it is as specific as a fingerprint. One look at the pedigree points me in the proper direction and guides me in devising a diet and disease-prevention strategies. An example of one person's pedigree is:

BLOOD TYPE	SECRETOR STATUS	NEG/POS	MN
O	Lewis a+ b– (non-secretor)	Rh–	MM

Another is:

BLOOD TYPE	SECRETOR STATUS	NEG/POS	MN
A	Lewis a– b+ (secretor)	Rh+	MN

If you wish to refine your program to this degree, you will find laboratories and other resources in the back of this book. However, don't get sidetracked from the main point: Knowing your ABO blood type alone will give you 90 percent of the information you need, and that should be your primary focus.

Resources: Getting Help

Dr. Peter D'Adamo is in private practice in Stamford, CT. For general information, to be put on a mailing list, or to comment on your own experiences with the Blood Type Diet, please use the P.O. box number or the Internet address.

PETER D'ADAMO, N.D.
2009 Summer St.
Stamford, CT 06905

P.O. Box 2106
Norwalk, CT 06852-2106

Materials Available

Visit Dr. D'Adamo's web site for the latest blood type news at. www.dadamo.com

For information regarding blood type–specific food supplements, home test kits, educational literature, and home blood typing kits, please contact:

NORTH AMERICAN PHARMACAL, INC.
17 High Street
Norwalk, CT 06851
877-ABO-TYPE (toll-free)
877-226-8973

Physicians wishing to apply the blood-typing system can order testing from:

DR. THOMAS KRUZEL, N.D., M.T.
800 SE 181st Ave
Gresham, OR 97233
(503) 667-1961

Naturopathic Physicians

Peter D'Adamo's father, who pioneered much of the initial research and clinical work on blood types, is still in practice. You may reach James D'Adamo, N.D., at:

44-46 Bridge St.
Portsmouth, NH 03801

To find a licensed naturopathic physician in your area, contact:

THE AMERICAN ASSOCIATION OF NATUROPATHIC PHYSICIANS
601 Valley St.
Suite 105
Seattle, WA 98109
(206) 298-0125

References

R ATHER THAN FILL THIS BOOK WITH ENDLESS FOOTNOTES, I'VE collected the most important influences on it and listed them here where they might be most easily referred to. They are grouped into several categories and listed alphabetically by author.

Blood types, general information

American Association of Blood Banks. *Technical Manual,* 10th ed. 1990.
D'Adamo, P. "Gut ecosystems III: The ABO and other polymorphic systems." *Townsend Ltr. for Doctors,* Aug. 1990.
Marcus, D. M. "The ABO and Lewis blood-group system." *New England J. Med.,* 280 (1969): 994–1005.

Diet and lifestyle

Atkins, R., and Herwood, R. W. *Dr. Atkins's Diet Revolution.* New York: Bantam, 1972.
D'Adamo, J. *The D'Adamo Diet.* Montreal: McGraw-Hill Ryerson, 1989.
———. *One Man's Food.* New York: Marek, 1980. (out of print).
Kushi, M., and Jack, A. *The Cancer Prevention Diet.* New York: St. Martin's, 1983.
Nomi, T., and Besher, A. *You Are Your Blood Type.* New York: Pocket, 1983.
Pritikin, N., and McGrady, P. *The Pritikin Program for Diet and Exercise.* New York: Grosset & Dunlap. 1979.
Schmid, R., *Traditional Foods Are Your Best Medicine.* New York: Ballantine, 1987.

Blood types and anthropology

Boyd, W. C. *Genetics and the Races of Man: An Introduction to Modern Physical Anthropology.* Boston: Little, Brown, 1950.

Brues, A. M. "Tests of blood group selection." *Amer. J. Forensic Medicine,* 1929: 287–89.

Childe, V. G. *Man Makes Himself.* London: Watts, 1936.

Coon, C. S. *The Races of Europe.* New York: Macmillan, 1939.

Gates, R. R. *Human Ancestry.* Cambridge, MA: Harvard University Press, 1948.

Hirszfeld, L., and Hirszfeld, H. *Lancet,* 2 (1919): 675.

Livingstone, F. R. "Natural selection disease and ongoing human evolution as illustrated by the ABO groups." Source unknown (copy in author's possession).

McNeil, W. H. *Plagues and Peoples.* New York: Doubleday/Anchor, 1975.

Mourant, A. E. *Blood Relations: Blood Groups and Anthropology.* Oxford, England: Oxford University Press, 1983.

———, Kopec, A. C., and Domaniewska-Sobczak, K. *Blood Groups and Disease,* Oxford England: Oxford University Press, 4th ed. 1984.

Muschel, L. "Blood groups, disease and selection." *Bacteriological Rev.,* 30, 2 (1966): 427–41.

Race, R. R., and Sanger, R. *Blood Groups in Man.* Oxford, England: Blackwell Scientific, 1975.

Sheppard, P. M. "Blood groups and natural selection." *Brit. Med. Bull.,* 15 (1959): 132–39.

Soulsby, E. H. L. "Antigen-antibody reactions in helminth infections." *Adv. Immunol.,* 2 (1962): 265–308.

Wyman, L. C., and Boyd, W. C. "Blood group determinations of prehistoric American Indians." *Amer. Anthropol.,* 39 (1937): 583–92.

———. "Human blood groups and anthropology." *Amer. Anthropol.,* 37 (1935): 181.

Blood types and lectins

D'Adamo, P. "Gut ecosystems II: Lectins and other mitogens." *Townsend Ltr. for Doctors,* 1991.

Freed, D. L. F. "Dietary lectins and disease." *Food Allergy and Intolerance,* 1987: 375–400.

————. "Lectins." *British Med. J.*, 290 (1985): 585–86.

Helm, R., and Froese, A. "Binding of receptors for IgE by various lectins." *Int. Arch. Allergy Appl. Immunology*, 65 (1981): 81–84.

Nachbar, M. S., et al. "Lectins in the U.S. diet: Isolation and characterization of a lectin from the tomato (*Lycopersicon esculentum*)." *J. Biol. Chem.*, 255 (1980): 2056–61.

Nachbar, M. S., et al. "Lectins in the U.S. diet: A survey of lectins in commonly consumed foods and a review of the literature." *Amer. J. Clin. Nut.*, 33 (1980): 233845.

Norn, S., et al. "Intrinsic asthma and bacterial histamine release via lectin effect." *Agents and Action*, 12, 2/3 (1983).

Sharon, N., and Halina, L. "The biochemistry of plant lectins (phytohemaglutinins A)." *Ann. Rev. Biochem.*, 42 (1973): 541–74.

————. "Lectins: Cell agglutinating and sugar-specific proteins." *Science*, 177 (1972): 949–59.

Shechter, Y. "Bound lectins that mimic insulin produce persistent insulin-like effects." *Endocrinology*, 113 (1983): 1921–26.

Triadou, N., and Audron, E. "Interaction of the brush border hydrolases of the human small intestine with lectins." *Digestion*, 27 (1983): 1–7.

Uhlendruck, G., et al. "Love to lectins: Personal history and priority hysterics." *Lectins and Glycoconjugates in Oncology*. New York: Springer-Verlag, date.

Uimer, A. J., et al. "Stimulation of colony formation and growth factor production of human lymphocytes by wheat germ lectin." *Immunology*, 47 (1982): 551–56.

Wagner, H., et al. "Immunostimulant action of polysaccharides (heteroglycans) from higher plants." *Arzneimittelforschung* 34 (1984): 659–61 (German abstract in English).

Waxdal, M. J. "Isolation, characterization and biological activities of five mitogens from pokeweed." *Biochemistry*, 13 (1974): 3671–75.

Zafrini, D., et al. "Inhibitory activity of cranberry juice on adherence of type 1 and type P fimbriated *E. coli* to eucaryotic cells." *Antimicrobial Agents and Chemotherapy*, 33 (1989): 92–98.

The Lectins: Properties, Functions and Applications in Biology and Medicine. New York: Harcourt Brace Jovanovich/Academic Press, 1986.

Disease associations with blood type

Addi, G. J. "Blood groups in acute rheumatism." *Scottish Med. J.*, 4 (1959): 547.

Aird, I., et al. "Blood groups in relation to peptic ulceration and carcinoma of the breast, colon, bronchus and rectum." *Brit. Med. J.*, 1954: 315–42.

Allan, T. M., and Dawson, A. A. "ABO blood groups and ischemic heart disease in men." *Brit. Heart J.*, 30 (1968): 377–82.

Billington, B. P. "Note on the distribution of ABO blood groups in bronchiectasis and portal cirrhosis." *Australian Ann. Med.*, 5 (1956): 20–22.

"Blood groups and the intestine" (editorial). *Lancet*, 7475 (Dec. 3, 1966).

Buchanan, J. A., and Higley, E. T. "The relationship of blood groups to disease." *Brit. J. Exper. Pathol.*, 2 (1921): 247–53.

Buckwalter, et al. "Ethnologic aspects of the ABO blood groups: Disease associations." *JAMA*, 1957: 327.

Buckwalter, et al. "ABO blood groups and disease." *JAMA*, 1956: 1210–4.

Camps, E. E., and Dodd, B. E. "Frequencies of secretors and non-secretors of ABH group substances among 1000 alcoholic patients." *Brit. Med. J.*, 4 (1969): 457–59.

———. "Increase in the incidence of non-secretors of ABH blood group substances among alcoholic patients." *Brit. Med. J.* 1 (1967): 30–31.

D'Adamo, P. "Blood types and diseases, a review." Clinical rounds presentation, Bastyr University 1982.

———. "Combination naturopathic treatment of primary biliary cirrhosis." *J. Naturopathic Med.*, 4, 1 (1993): 24–25.

———, and Zampieron, E. "Does ABO bias in natural immunity imply an innate difference in T-cell response?" *J. Naturopathic Med.*, 2 (1991): 11–17.

"Blood groups and susceptibility to disease: A review." *Brit. J. Prev. Soc. Med.*, 11 (1957): 107–25.

Fraser Roberts, J. A. "Some associations between blood types and disease." *Brit. Med. Bull.*, 15 (1959): 129–33.

Harris, R., et al. "Vaccine virus and human blood group A substance." *Acta Genetica*, 13 (1963): 44–57.

Havlik, R., et al. "Blood groups and coronary heart disease" (letter). *Lancet*, Aug. 2, 1969: 269–70.

Hein, O. H., et al. "Alcohol consumption, Lewis phenotypes, and the risk of ischemic heart disease." *Lancet*, Feb. 13, 1993: 392–96.

"An insight is gained on how ulcers develop." *The New York Times*, Dec. 17, 1993.

Koskins, L. C., et al. "Degradation of blood group antigens in human colon ecosystems." *J. Clin. Invest*, 57 (1976): 63–73.

Langman, M. J. S. et al. "ABO and Lewis blood groups and serum cholesterol." *Lancet*, Sept. 20, 1969: 607–9.

Lim, W., et al. "Association of secretor status and rheumatic fever in 106 families." *Amer. J. Epidemiology*, 82 (1965): 103–11.

McConnell, R. B., et al. "Blood groups in diabetes mellitis." *Brit. Med. J.*, 1 (1956): 772–76.

McDuffie and Hart. "The behavior in the Coombs test of anti-A and anti-B produced by immunization with various blood group specific substances and by heterospecific pregnancy." *J. Immunology*, 77 (1956): 61–71.

Martin, N. G., et al. "Do the MN and JK systems influence environmental variability in serum lipid levels?" *Clinical Genetics*, 24 (1983): 1–14.

Myrianthopolous, N. C., et al. "Relation of blood groups and secretor factor to amyotrophic lateral sclerosis." *Amer. J. Human Genetics*, 19 (1967): 607–16.

"O! My aching stomach!" Witby *Republican*, Dec. 12, 1993.

Ratner, et al. "ABO group uropathogens and urinary tract infection." *Amer. J. Med. Sci.*, 292 (1986): 84–92.

Roath, S., et al. "Transient acquired blood group B antigen associated with diverticular bowel disease." *Acta Haematologica*, 77 (1987): 188–90.

Springer, G. F. "Relation of blood group active plant substances to human blood groups." *Acta Haem.*, 20 (1958): 147–55.

———, and Horton, R. E. "Erythrocyte sensitization by blood group specific bacterial antigens." *J. Gen. Physio.*, 47 (1964): 1229–49.

Struthers, D. "ABO groups of infants and children dying in the west of Scotland (1949–51)." *Brit. J. Soc. Prev. Med.*, 5 (1951): 223–28.

Young, V. M., Gillem, H. G., and Akeroyd, J. H. "Sensitization of infant red cells by bacterial polysaccharides of *E. coli* during enteritis." *J. Ped.*, 60 (1962): 172–76.

Blood types and cancer

Aird, I., et al. "ABO blood groups and cancer of the esophagus, cancer of the pancreas and pituitary adenoma." *Brit. Med. J.,* 1 (1960): 1163–66.

Aird, E., et al. "Blood groups in relationship to peptic ulceration, and carcinoma of the colon, rectum, breast and bronchus." *Brit. Med. J.,* 2 (1954): 315–21.

Aird, E., et al. "Relationship between ABO group and cancer of the stomach." *Brit. Med. J.,* 1 (1954): 799–801.

Bazeed, M. A., et al. "Effect of lectins on KK-47 bladder cancer cell line." *Urology,* 32, 2 (1988): 133–35.

Boland, C. R. "Searching for the face of cancer." *J. Clin. Gastroenterology,* 10, 6 (1988): 599–604.

Brooks, S. A. "Predictive value of lectin binding on breast cancer recurrence and survival." *Lancet,* May 9, 1987: 1054–56.

————, and Leathem, A. J. C. "Prediction of lymph node involvement in breast cancer by detection of altered glycosylation in the primary tumor." *Lancet,* 8759, 338 (1991): 71–74.

Cameron, C., et al. "Acquisition of a B-like antigen by red blood cells." *Brit. Med. J.,* July 11, 1959: 29–34.

D'Adamo, P. "Possible alteration of ABO blood group observed in non-Hodgkin's lymphoma." *J. Naturopath. Med.,* 1 (1990): 39–43.

Dahiya, R., et al. "ABH blood group antigen expression, synthesis and degradation in human colonic adenocarcinoma cell lines." *Cancer Res.,* 49, 16 (1989): 4550–56.

Dahiya, R., et al. "ABH blood group antigen synthesis in human colonic adenocarcinoma cell lines" (meeting abstract). *Proc. Ann. Mtg. Amer. Assoc. Cancer Res.,* 30 (1989): A1405.

Davis, D. L., et al. "Medical hypothesis: Xenoestrogens as preventable causes of breast cancer." *Environ. Health Persp.,* 101, 5, (1993): 372–777.

Feinmesser, R., et al. "Lectin binding characteristics of laryngeal cancer." *Otolaryngeal Head Neck Surgery,* 100, 3 (1989): 207–9.

Fenlon, S., et al. "*Helix pomatia* and *Ulex europeus* lectin binding in human breast carcinoma." *J. Pathology,* 152 (1987): 169–76.

Kvist, E., et al. "Relationship between blood groups and tumors of the upper urinary tract." *Scand. J. Urol. Nephrol.,* 22, 4 (1988): 289–91.

Langkilde, N. C., et al. "Binding of wheat and peanut lectins to human transitional cell carcinoma." *Cancer,* 64, 4 (1989): 849–53.

Lemon, H. "Clinical and experimental aspects of anti-mammary carcinogenic activity of estriol." *Front. Hormone Res.,* 5 (1978): 155–73.

———. "Pathophysiological considerations in the treatment of menopausal patients with estrogens: The role of estriol in the prevention of mammary carcinoma." *Acta Endocrin. Supp.,* 233 (1980): 17–27.

Marth, C., and Daxenbichiler, G. "Peanut agglutinin inhibits proliferation of cultured breast cancer cells." *Oncology,* 45 (1988): 47–50.

Morecki, S., et al. "Removal of breast cancer cells by soybean agglutinin in experimental model for purging human marrow." *Canc. Res.,* 48 (1988): 4573–77.

Motzer, R. J., et al. "Blood group related antigens in human germ cell tumors." *Cancer Res.,* 48, 18 (1988): 5342–47.

Murata, K., et al. "Expression of blood group related antigens ABH, Lewis a, Lewis b, Lewis x, Lewis y, Ca19-9 and CSLEX1 in early cancer, intestinal metaplasia and uninvolved mucosa of the stomach." *Amer. J. Clin. Path.,* 98 (1992): 67–75.

Osborne, R. H., and DeGeorge, F. V. "ABO blood groups and neoplastic disease of the ovary." *Amer. J. Human Genetics,* 15 (1963): 380–88.

Renton, P. H., et al. "Red cells of all four ABO groups in a case of leukemia." *Brit. Med. J.,* Feb. 2, 1962: 294–97.

Roberts, T. E., et al. "Blood groups and lung cancer" (letter). *Brit. J. Cancer,* 58, 2 (1988): 278.

Romodanov, S. A., et al. "Efficacy of chemo and immunochemistry in neuro-oncological patients with different ABO system blood group." *ZH-Vopr-Neirkhiir Im Nn Burdenko,* 53/1, 17–20 (1989).

Stachura, J., et al. "Blood group antigens in the distribution of pancreatic cancer." *Folia Histochem. Cytobiol.,* 27, 1 (1989): 49–55.

Springer, G., et al. "Blood group MN antigens and precursors in normal and malignant human breast glandular tissue." *J. Nat. Cancer Instit.,* 54, 2 (1975): 335–39.

Springer, G., et al. "T/Tn antigen vaccine is effective and safe in preventing recurrence of advanced breast cancer." *Cancer Detection and Prevention* (in press, 1993).

Tryggvadottir, L., et al. "Familial and sporadic breast cancer cases in Iceland: A comparison related to ABO blood groups and risk of bilateral breast cancer." *Inter. J. Cancer,* 42, 4 (1988): 499–501.

Tzingounis, V. A., et al. "Estriol in the management of menopause."
JAMA, 239, 16 (1978): 1638.

Wolf, G. T., et al. "A9 and ABH antigen expression predicts outcome in
head and neck cancer." *Proc. Ann. Mtg. Amer. Assoc. Cancer Res.*, 30
(1989): A902.

Survey:

Be a Part of the Blood Type Revolution

THE BLOOD TYPE REVOLUTION CONTINUES FOR ALL those who make the Blood Type Diet a part of their life. I am continuing to research the special conditions that the Blood Type Diets address, as well as the particular ancestries that seem linked to certain blood types and conditions.

I am very eager for your input. After you have followed the Blood Type Diet for at least three months or more, I welcome a report of what happened to you. I am also interested in hearing about adaptations you have made in menus and recipes that may be of use to others.

Your involvement in this work is an important contribution to the lives and health of others. Thank you for joining the revolution!

Part I: Background

Age ____
Sex ____ M ____ F

Blood Type   ____ O   ____ A   ____ B   ____ AB

If you know your subgroup, include the information here:

Rhesus Group   ____ Rh+   ____ Rh–

Secretor Status   ____ secretor   ____ non-secretor

MN Blood Group   ____ MM   ____ MN   ____ NN

Family Blood Type Tree

If you can find out the following blood types, it will enhance your understanding of the significance of your blood type legacy.

FATHER'S SIDE   **MOTHER'S SIDE**

your grandfather ____   your grandfather ____
your grandmother ____   your grandmother ____
your father ____   your mother ____

(if applicable, your spouse:)

FATHER'S SIDE   **MOTHER'S SIDE**

your grandfather ____   your grandfather ____
your grandmother ____   your grandmother ____
your father ____   your mother ____

you ____   your spouse ____
your children ____   ____   ____   ____   ____

Your father's ancestry: _____

Your spouse's father's ancestry: _____

Your mother's ancestry: _____

Your spouse's mother's ancestry: _____

Are there particular illnesses or diseases that run in your or your spouse's family? Yes ____   No ____
If yes, please elaborate.

Part II: Your Personal History

Do you have current medical conditions for which you are receiving treatment? Yes _____   No _____
If yes, please elaborate.

Do you have past medical conditions for which you have received treatment? Yes _____   No _____
If yes, please elaborate.

Have you ever had surgery? Yes _____   No _____
If yes, please elaborate.

Are you now or have you ever been on medications? Yes _____
No _____
If yes, please elaborate.

Would you consider yourself: _____ overweight
_____ average   _____ underweight

What is your profession? _____

Would you consider it   _____ high stress   _____ medium stress
_____ low stress

Would you consider yourself:
_____ an exceptionally heavy exerciser
_____ a regular exerciser
_____ a light exerciser
_____ no exercise to speak of

If you exercise regularly, what kinds of exercise do you enjoy?

What is your typical diet? List the foods you commonly eat.

Have you ever tried a special diet program? If so, what was the program and why did you start it? What were the results?

Part III: Your Experience with
the Blood Type Diet

Why did you decide to try the Blood Type Diet? Give as much detail as you can. For example, did you or a member of your family have a medical condition that you thought could be helped? Did you decide after reading the book that this approach offered the opportunity to take further control of the choices you make now that will affect you in the future?

How long have you been on the Blood Type Diet? ____

What were the most difficult adjustments for you to make?

Have you also followed the exercise recommendations? If so, what have you noticed about your stress level and general state of conditioning? If you changed radically from the exercise style you were used to (i.e., from running to yoga), describe that change. Do you feel it's worked for you, or not?

What has been your overall experience with the Blood Type Diet?

(If applicable) Have your partner and your children also tried the Blood Type Diet? If so, what has been their experience?

Have you come up with any terrific recipes or alternative foods that have made the Blood Type Diet work for you? If possible, please enclose them.

Have you found good ways to balance the needs of family members with different blood types? Please share them.

Do you have any final observations about the value of the Blood Type Diet that you would like to share? I welcome comments that might lead me to further clarify my work.

(optional)
Name: _____
Address: _____
City: _____   State: _____   Zip _____
Phone: _____

Would you be willing to be contacted about your experiences with the Blood Type Diet? Yes _____   No _____

Would you like to be put on a mailing list to receive updated information on blood type research and therapies?
Yes _____   No _____

Are you interested in receiving information on ordering home blood-testing kits? Yes _____   No _____

Thank you!

Return this survey to:
  PETER D'ADAMO, N.D.
  Survey
  P.O. Box 2106
  Norwalk, CT 06852-2106